FIRST PLACE BIBLE STUDY

LIVING *the* LEGACY

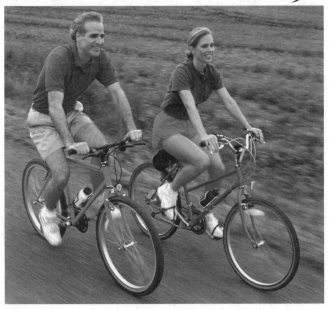

Gospel Light

FIRST PLACE™

PUBLISHING STAFF

William T. Greig, Chairman
Kyle Duncan, Publisher
Dr. Elmer L. Towns, Senior Consulting Publisher
Pam Weston, Senior Editor
Patti Pennington Virtue, Associate Editor
Jeff Kempton, Editorial Assistant
Hilary Young, Editorial Assistant
Bayard Taylor, M.Div., Senior Editor, Biblical and Theological Issues
Barbara LeVan Fisher, Packaging Concept and Design
Samantha A. Hsu, Cover and Internal Designer

CAUTION

The information contained in this book is intended to be solely informational and educational. It is assumed that the First Place participant will consult a medical or health professional before beginning this or any other weight-loss or physical-fitness program.

CONTENTS

FOREWORD

My introduction to Bible study came when I joined First Place in March of 1981. I had been in church since I was a small child, but the extent of my study of the Bible had been reading my Sunday School quarterly on Saturday night. On Sunday morning, I would listen to my Sunday School teacher as she taught God's Word to me. During the worship service, I would listen to our pastor as he taught God's Word to me. Digging out the truths of the Bible for myself had frankly never entered my mind.

Perhaps you are right where I was back in 1981. If so, you are in for a blessing you never dreamed possible. As you start studying the truths of the Bible for yourself, you will see God begin to open your understanding of His Word. Bible study is one of the nine commitments of the First Place program. The First Place Bible studies are designed to be done on a daily basis. Each day's study will take approximately 15 to 20 minutes to complete, but you will be discovering the deep truths of God's Word as you work through each week's study.

There are many in-depth Bible studies on the market. The First Place Bible studies are not designed for the purpose of in-depth study. They are designed to be used in conjunction with the other eight commitments of the program to bring balance into our lives. Our desire is for each member to begin having a personal quiet time with God each day. This time alone with God should include a time of prayer, Bible reading and Bible study. Having a quiet time is a daily discipline that will bring the rich rewards of balance, something we all need.

A part of each week's study is the Bible memory verse for the week. You will find a CD at the back of this Bible study that contains all 10 of the memory verses for the study set to music. The CD has an upbeat tempo suitable for use when exercising. The songs help you to memorize the verses easily and retain them for future reference. If you memorize Scripture as you study, God will use His Word to transform your life.

Almost every First Place member I have talked with about the program says, "The weight loss is wonderful, but the most important thing I have received from my association with First Place is learning to study God's Word."

God bless you as you begin this exciting journey toward a balanced life. God will richly bless your efforts to give Him first place in your life. Remember Matthew 6:33: "But seek first his kingdom and his righteousness, and all these things will be given to you as well."

Carole Lewis
First Place National Director

INTRODUCTION

The First Place Bible studies were developed to be used in conjunction with the First Place weight-loss program. However, the studies could also be used by anyone who desires to learn more about God's Word and His will, with the added bonus of learning more about living a healthy lifestyle.

A Balanced Life

First Place is a Christ-centered health program, emphasizing balance in the physical, mental, emotional and spiritual areas of life. The First Place program is meant to be a daily process. As we learn to keep Christ first in our lives, we will find that He is the One who satisfies our hunger and our every need.

God's Word contains guidelines for maintaining our physical well-being, equipping us mentally to make right choices, providing emotional stability to handle everyday circumstances as well as crisis situations, and growing spiritually as we deepen our relationship with Him.

The Nine Commitments

The First Place program has nine commitments that will help you draw closer to the Lord and aid you in establishing a solid, consistent and healthy Christian life. Each commitment is a necessary and important part of the goal of First Place to help you become healthier and stronger in all areas of your life—living the abundant life He has planned for each of us. To help you achieve growth in all four areas, First Place asks you to keep these nine commitments:

1. Attendance
2. Encouragement
3. Prayer
4. Bible reading
5. Scripture memory verse
6. Bible study
7. Live-It plan
8. Commitment Record
9. Exercise

The Components

There are six distinct components to this Bible study to aid you in bringing balance to your life. These components include the 10-week Bible study, 6 Wellness Worksheets, 2 weeks of menu plans, the leader's discussion guide, 13 Commitment Records and the Scripture Memory Music CD.

The Bible Study

Each week of each 10-week Bible study is divided into five daily assignments with Days 6 and 7 set aside for reflections on the week's lesson. The following guidelines will help make your study more enjoyable and profitable:

- Set aside 15 to 20 minutes each day to complete the daily assignment. It's best not to attempt to complete a week's worth of Bible study in one day.
- Pray before each day's study and ask God to give you understanding and a teachable heart.
- Keep in mind that the ultimate goal of Bible study is not for knowledge only but also for application and a changed life.
- First Place suggests using the *New International Version* of the Bible to complete the studies.
- Don't feel anxious if you can't seem to find the *correct* answer. Many times the Word will speak differently to different people, depending upon where they are in their walk with God and the season of life they are experiencing.
- Be prepared to discuss with your fellow First Place members what you learned that week through your study.

Wellness Worksheets

The informative and interactive Wellness Worksheets have been developed by Dr. Jody Wilkinson of the Cooper Institute in Dallas, Texas. These worksheets are intended to help you understand and achieve balance in all four areas of your life: physical, mental, emotional and spiritual. Your leader will assign specific worksheets as At-Home Assignments throughout the 13-week session.

Menu Plans

The two-week menu plans were developed especially for First Place by Chef Scott Wilson. Each menu is meant to simplify meal planning and include food exchanges. These meals are based on the MasterCook software that uses a database of over 6,000 food items, which was prepared using United States Department of Agriculture (USDA) publications and information from food manufacturers.

Leader's Discussion Guide

This discussion guide is provided to help the First Place leader guide a group through this Bible study. It provides information for the leader to prepare for each weekly group meeting.

Personal Weight Record

The Personal Weight Record is for the member to use to keep a record of weight loss. After the weigh-in at each week's meeting, the member will record any loss or gain on the chart.

Commitment Records

Thirteen Commitment Records (CRs) are provided in the back of this Bible study. For your convenience these have been printed on perforated paper so that you may easily remove them from the book and carry them with you through each week as you keep your First Place commitments. Directions for filling out the CRs precedes those pages.

Scripture Memory CD

Since Scripture memory music is such a vital part of the First Place program, the Scripture Memory Music CD for this study is included in the back inside cover. The verses for this study are set to music that can be listened to as you work, play or travel. The CD can be an effective tool as you exercise since the first verse is set to music with a warm-up tempo, the next eight verses are set to workout tempo, and the music of the last verse can be used for a cooldown.

A DIVINE INHERITANCE

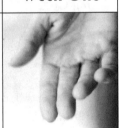

MEMORY VERSE
He chose us in him before the creation of the world
to be holy and blameless in his sight.
Ephesians 1:4

Returning from the Christmas holidays, a struggling college student arrived in her sparse dormitory room to find an envelope addressed to her from a large law firm. The letter had been delivered by certified mail and signed for by her roommate, so she knew it must be important. Still, she couldn't imagine why a law firm would want to contact her.

The envelope indeed held an important document: a letter explaining that the law firm had been instructed by the student's late father to transfer her inheritance into her name on her twenty-first birthday, a birthday she had celebrated over the holidays. The student was unaware of any inheritance; her father had died when she was very young, and no one had mentioned a will in all those years. Although the financial arrangements were complex, the young woman came to understand very quickly that she was rich—undeniably rich.

Like this young student, *you* have an inheritance as a child of your heavenly Father. Unlike the student, your inheritance is available right now; there is no waiting period. As a joint heir with Christ, you are entitled to everything the Father has to give, but wealth brings responsibility. In this week's study, we will explore the blessings and responsibilities of our inheritance in Christ.

DAY 1: *Special Gifts*

The apostle Paul knew he was an heir to the greatest fortune mankind has ever known. He desperately wanted to share this knowledge with you.

His desire was for you to know that you, too, are a blessed child of the King of kings.

>> Read Ephesians 1:1-14. List the gifts we receive as children of the living God.

Do you feel like a rich beneficiary as you read this passage? Some might think, *I know I have an inheritance waiting for me in heaven, but wouldn't it be nice to enjoy some of it in this life?* The inheritance you have received is not on layaway; it is given for your earthly enjoyment today. God intended for you to have a more abundant life than you can ever imagine.

As you meditate on the different aspects of your inheritance, think about how you see evidence of each of those gifts in your personal life. The first of these gifts is that you are *blessed*. We will look more at the implication of this gift in tomorrow's study.

>> Reread Ephesians 1:3 and list the spiritual blessings you have experienced.

Every spiritual blessing—from God's agape love to Christ's sacrificial death and from His glorious resurrection to the gift of the Holy Spirit—is from above. Your list could be endless! These blessings are from Christ who now reigns in heaven. Every day make a list of things for which you are thankful that day. Thank God for the blessings He gives you each day.

Heavenly Father, You give me so many blessings that my heart overflows with praise and thanksgiving.

Dear Lord, thank You for the rich inheritance that is mine through Your Son, my Lord Jesus Christ.

Day 2: *Blessed*

The ageless book of Ephesians is a living will and testament from God to His precious children. Your heavenly Father has given you an inheritance based on nothing you have done. Like the college student in this week's introduction, you are the recipient because of a death in the family. Through the death of Christ, and no other way, you have wealth you could never have earned. Yet it cost you nothing—and Christ everything! What a blessing!

Paul knew that our being God's heirs would invite attacks by our enemy, Satan, who does not want us to enjoy the benefits of our rich inheritance.

➳ What is the dilemma faced by all Christians that is described in Galatians 5:17?

Perhaps you joined First Place to combat this very dilemma: the flesh wars against the Spirit in you. The Spirit reminds you that your body is God's temple and deserves special treatment.

➳ What does 1 Corinthians 6:19-20 tell you about your body?

Although your body is not your own to do with as you will, the flesh convinces you that certain harmful things will bring happiness. It lures you to lead a sedentary lifestyle rather than one of physical fitness. Or it entices you to indulge in foods that are harmful to you.

➳ What is the encouraging promise found in 1 Corinthians 10:13?

➤ According to James 1:12, what specific action has God promised to bless?

God promises to bless you when you struggle against temptation rather than giving in to it. In the battle against unhealthy living, you will gain strength in areas where you are tempted to veer from God's will as you learn to depend on Him for victory.

➤ List one blessing that comes from withstanding temptation in your commitment to living a disciplined lifestyle.

 Heavenly Father, help me to overcome the temptations that may come into my life today. I claim Your promise to give me a way of escape.

Dear Lord, thank You for giving me the power to overcome my enemy and claim victory in Your name.

DAY 3: *Chosen and Holy*

When friends play childhood games, some children are rarely chosen first—and some not at all. You can be sure that your heavenly Father wants you on His team. You really rate with Him. The second blessing is that you are *chosen*.

God chose you because He loves you. Even before He created the world, He knew about you and developed a plan to save you and give you eternal life.

➤ Reread the memory verse, Ephesians 1:4, and complete the following statement:

God has chosen you to be_____and

_____.

➤ Holiness is the third gift of inheritance. Since God has chosen you to live in a holy and blameless manner, what lifestyle change(s) do you need to make?

Did you list such things as getting more sleep at night, watching what you eat, exercising more or spending more time in prayer and Bible study?

➤ After reading 1 Peter 1:13-16, list ways you can demonstrate holy living.

A blameless life seems impossible to attain and can discourage us from pursuing holiness. Remember that when God looks at you, He sees Christ's righteousness and not your own unrighteousness. However, God expects your willing cooperation in His efforts to make you more Christlike. If you are totally His, living a holy, blameless life will be your desire. Being holy involves completely belonging to Christ. It involves giving Him first place!

➤ How does the act of being holy impact your daily life? Put a check by the activities that result from having a heart totally committed to Him.

☐ Strive for a healthy lifestyle

☐ Look for ways to minister to others

☐ Lecture people about their sins

☐ Live so that people see Christ in me

☐ Boast when I accomplish a goal

If your heart is wholly His, every area of your life will be affected—even the area of healthy living.

Thank You, Holy Father, for choosing me to be one of Your disciples and for giving me my salvation full and free.

Dear Lord, help me to demonstrate my gratitude to You as I seek to live a holy life that is pleasing to You.

DAY 4: *Predestined*

The fourth gift of our inheritance is that we are *predestined*. Our lives are in God's powerful hands—not in the grip of capricious fate. Nothing that happens to you is a surprise to God. Think about it! He knows the issues that spurred you to participate in First Place.

➣ Consider Psalm 139:1-16; what is the blessing found in verses 7-12?

➣ How do you feel when you learn that God, Creator of this massive universe, knows and cares about even the smallest details of your life?

☐ It's impossible; God can't possibly care about the events of my daily life.

☐ I'm not worthy of this kind of care.

☐ I feel loved just thinking about it.

☐ Other _____

This is one of the most reassuring of the many psalms of David. How wonderfully and fearfully are you made. God knows every muscle, sinew, bone and cell of your body.

He provided for you before you were born. He sent Jesus to be your Savior so that you could have a restored relationship with Him. He has protected you and provided for you. He has provided the First Place program to help you take care of His creation. God is at work now in helping you to take care of what He provides for you. By taking care of His creation, you honor Him.

➣ According to Romans 8:28-30, for what purpose does God predestine you?

These verses show us God's eternal and unfailing purpose through His Word and His Son, Jesus Christ. You are to be conformed to the likeness of Christ. What a challenge for you as you honor God. If you ask Him, God will reveal to you the Christlike qualities you are to cultivate. In this you will honor Him in the way you talk, live and act.

Father God, thank You for the wonderful creation You made in me. I stand in awe of Your mighty power and Your unconditional love for me.

Lord Jesus, help me today to honor You in everything I do, so others may see Your love and mercy through me.

DAY 5: *Adopted and Forgiven*

Adoptive parents take a child into their home and give him or her all the rights and privileges of being their biological child. Although you did nothing to deserve it, God adopted you into His family of faith. Today you will look at the fifth and sixth gifts of inheritance, *adopted* and *forgiven*. Read or recite from memory John 3:16.

➤ What do you receive when you are adopted into God's family?

When you think about your vast inheritance, treasure the gift of eternal life. It cost you nothing; it cost Christ His life. Why did He do it? Because He loves you. Eternal life is yours because of God's willingness to forgive.

➤ According to Psalm 103:12, how far has God removed your sins from you?

If you look on a map or globe, you might pinpoint the North and South Poles. They are geographical locations. But can you find poles labeled East and West? Can you measure the distance between them? No. So you can never measure how far away God places your sin. Your transgressions of the past are no more in God's eyes.

➤ According to Romans 6:23, what payment do your sins deserve?

➤ What gift did God give you instead?

Your wrong acts merit death, but Christ took your penalty. Forgiveness is God's gracious act of forgetting every sin for which you repent and claim His forgiveness. God does not look to the past; He looks to your future. You are a forgiven child of God. What an inheritance!

➤ The following is a list of the blessings of your inheritance through Christ. Write next to each blessing what each one means to you.

1. Blessed

2. Chosen

3. Holy

4. Predestined

5. Adopted

6. Forgiven

These gifts of your inheritance place you above the wealthiest of this world. This inheritance doesn't buy earthly possessions, but it gives you possession of eternal life through Jesus Christ. Nothing is more valuable than that.

Thank You, Father God, for adopting me into Your family and giving me the inheritance of eternal life through Jesus Christ, Your beloved Son.

Heavenly Father, You took my sin away, and I now commit my life to You, to live the abundant life You offer me.

DAY 6: *Reflections*

On the last two days of each week's study, you will reflect on your memory verse and what it can mean to you. In addition, you will learn more about memorizing Scripture and praying by using the Word of God.

This week you have learned how God chose you before the creation of the world to be holy and blameless in His sight. Yes, He chose you to be His child, but not everyone becomes a child of God. How can that be? God gave each person a free will. This means you must also choose Him. God's plan is to have every man, woman and child inherit His kingdom, but you must choose to do so.

God's blessings and love are available to all, but not all choose to accept what God so freely offers. Your salvation is a special gift, and God paid a tremendous price for that gift. He paid for it with the death of His Son, Jesus Christ. Paul knew he was the heir to the greatest fortune mankind could ever have. So, dear one, are you.

Because you are so special to God, He wants to know you in an intimate relationship of love. He wants only what is best for you. He has a wonderful path for you, but it is up to you to seek His will for your life.

The way to know God intimately is through His Word. You have the Bible to tell you all about God and what He has done, is doing and will do in your life. The Bible is your "sword of the Spirit" (Ephesians 6:17) to help you win the war against sin. Scripture memory is the key to unlocking the treasure of your inheritance. Begin with the memory verse each week and marvel at the beauty of God's blessing for you.

Planting God's Word in your heart will help you understand the wealth of the inheritance God has for you on this earth. Dip into the riches He provides and find jewels of love and wisdom beyond comparison.

Holy God, I enter Your gates with thanksgiving and Your courts with praise; I give thanks to You and praise Your name (see Psalm 100:4).

O Lord, whatever I do in word or deed, I do it all in the name of the Lord Jesus Christ and give thanks to You, God my Father, through Him (see Colossians 3:17).

I give thanks, Father God, for the inheritance that can never perish, spoil or fade away and is kept in heaven for me (see 1 Peter 1:4).

DAY 7: *Reflections*

Scripture memory is a commitment you make when you join First Place. Each week you have one verse to memorize. This may seem an impossible task, but you are given resources to help make the task easier for you. You have a CD with all the memory verses set to music and you have the *Walking in the Word* book with all the verses within easy reach. Listen to your CD or tape in the car, at home, during exercise or on the job in place of a radio. Practice by reading/writing the Scripture verse each day.

Why memorize Scripture? What's its purpose in my life? Several good purposes come to mind. Each will be discussed during this study. Today the first purpose is to help you handle difficult situations. When you have God's words written in your heart, you are equipped to handle any situation you may face. Knowing that you can do all things through Christ (see Philippians 4:13) and that He will never desert you or forsake you (see Hebrews 13:5) enables you to walk through tough situations with peace and courage.

Praying God's Word by Beth Moore is an excellent resource to use in memorizing and using Scripture to pray. Her book will be used as a reference throughout the Bible studies in First Place. She teaches us how to overcome any and every situation through Scripture and prayer. She reinforces the discipline of memorizing God's Word.[1]

If Scripture memory is new to you, focus on your memory verse as a place to begin. Write it several times and repeat it aloud each time you write it. Remember to use the resources provided by First Place. The more you practice, the easier it will become. Tiger Woods may have been born with athletic abilities, but he didn't become a champion without practice, practice and more practice. Champions train for a lifetime to reach their goals. Start your training today as you memorize the verse for this week.

The following are verses that are easy to memorize and can be used as a focus for your thoughts during your prayer time:

Father God, thank You for loving this world so much that You gave Your one and only Son so that whoever believes on Him shall not perish but will have eternal life (see John 3:16).

Heavenly Father, I know that in all things You work for the good of those who love You and have been called according to Your purpose (see Romans 8:28).

Holy Lord, send Your peace that transcends all understanding to guard my heart and my mind in Christ Jesus (see Philippians 4:7).

O Lord God, thank You for choosing me in You before the creation of the world to be holy and blameless in Your sight (see Ephesians 1:4).

Note
1. Beth Moore, *Praying God's Word* (Nashville, TN: Broadman and Holman, 2000).

GROUP PRAYER REQUESTS   TODAY'S DATE:_____

NAME	REQUEST	RESULTS

GRACE STILL SO AMAZING

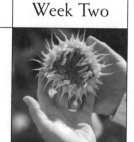

MEMORY VERSE

By grace you have been saved, through faith—
and this not from yourselves, it is a gift of God—
not by works, so that no one can boast.
Ephesians 2:8-9

After overhearing his son fire an employee for misconduct, the father quizzed his son. "You are such a patient and loving father to your daughters," he began. "Why couldn't you have treated that employee with the same forgiveness and offered him another chance?" The son replied by explaining that his employees were under the law but his daughters were under grace.

What do you think the son meant by his statement? What is the difference between law and grace? Many people do not grow up in a grace-filled environment. This week you will focus on God's grace as part of your inheritance as a child of the King.

DAY 1: *Believe God's Promises*

Last week's study was an overview of the various aspects of your inheritance: You are blessed, chosen, holy, predestined, adopted and forgiven. You may be awestruck by such blessings and be tempted to ask, "Why does the Lord God give me such a divine inheritance?" Does He actually have the authority to forgive you, to bless you, to choose you, to adopt you and to wipe your sins away? God has the authority because He acts according to who He is to the world—Creator and Sovereign—and who He is to you—your Father.

➤ What do Genesis 1:1 and Isaiah 66:1-2 say about God, who He is and by what authority He acts?

✤ Who does John say Jesus is in John 1:3?

✤ According to 1 Corinthians 15:27-28, what is Jesus' role?

Yes, Jesus is the One by whom and for whom all things were made. He was an active part of the creation process. Everything was put under Christ and is subject to God who is all in all. As God's only Son, Jesus is the firstfruits of our inheritance (see 1 Corinthians 15:23). Jesus is your guarantee that God will deliver all He promises!

✤ Which of the following do you have difficulty believing? Check all that apply.

    ☐ God chose me because He loves me.

    ☐ ˈ am fully forgiven.

    ☐ God sees me as holy because of Christ's righteousness.

    ☐ None of the above.

Do you believe the promises of God? Unbelief results from lack of faith.

✤ What are the promises and assurances found in Colossians 1:15-17 and Hebrews 11:3,39?

These verses affirm who God is and why He has the authority to leave you His matchless inheritance. He is Creator and Sustainer of all—including you!

 Father God, I praise Your name as the Creator of the universe and of all things that live and breathe, including me.

Heavenly Father, I humbly accept Your matchless inheritance and praise Your name above all the heavens.

DAY 2: *Accept God's Gift*

A middle-school counselor wasn't impressed by a student's past grades, but he believed the boy could excel if put into a challenging environment. The counselor, with the approval of the principal, called the boy to his office and told him, "I'm going to enroll you in an honors class next fall. Your grades don't qualify you, but I believe you can do the work." Prompted by the gracious act of a man who believed in him, the boy went on to academic success.

Grace is the utter generosity of God given to you as an adopted child, even though as a sinner you don't deserve it.

➣ Use the memory verse, Ephesians 2:8-9, to complete the following statement:

Salvation comes as a result of_____not from
_____.

You have not earned salvation. Like the middle-school student in the honors class, your performance in life has not qualified you for the gift of salvation. Grace has made this free gift of salvation possible for you. Your part is simply to accept God's grace.

➣ According to Romans 5:8, how did God show His love for you as a sinner?

On the cross God offered His most precious possession—His Son—as payment for your sins in order to restore your relationship with a holy God. Grace is the means by which God gives the sinner an undeserved inheritance. He paid your debt in full!

➣ Are you the recipient of God's grace? If so, how can you show your gratitude this week?

God paid a tremendous price for your life.

➤ According to 1 Corinthians 6:19-20, what is your responsibility toward the gift you've received?

➤ What are some ways you can honor God with your body?

Thank You, Father for bringing me into Your kingdom through Your Son, the Lord Jesus Christ.

Heavenly Father, I ask You today to give me an attitude of thanksgiving and praise for Your abundant grace.

DAY 3: *Have Great Expectations*

In the Charles Dickens novel *Great Expectations*, the young boy Pip had great expectations for his future. However, his life didn't turn out as he had expected. Parents often have great expectations for their new baby. Will he or she be a great athlete, sing solos or excel in school? Sometimes children take a different path and fall short of their parent's expectations. God has expectations for you. With His help, you will attain them. If you ignore God's guidance and leadership, you too will fall short of what you can be through Him.

➤ What are God's expectations for you, according to Colossians 1:10?

➣ Read Ephesians 2:12-13; then check the words that best describe you before Christ came into your life.

☐ Separate from Christ   ☐ Without God
☐ Without hope   ☐ Far away

Did you check all of them? This describes you without God in your life. God did not create you to be subject to the natural desires of your sinful nature. He had much higher expectations for you.

➣ How are believers described in Ephesians 2:19-22?

God desires and expects your walk to be different now that you are a new person in Christ.

➣ How should knowing you are a holy temple in which God lives affect the way you treat your body?

➣ What impact do the ways of the world now have on you? Circle a number on the following scale that indicates where you stand in relation to being controlled by messages from the world.

1	2	3	4	5

Not affected   Greatly affected

Some of the world's messages may include: eat all you want; gratify your desires; allow your emotions to dictate your choices; indulge in harmful habits; if it feels good, do it.

Maybe you once had high expectations for your new life in Christ but now feel you are failing to live up to those expectations. Satan is producing those feelings; he can gain control in a small area and use that to make you feel unworthy, even useless in God's kingdom. Good news! God can regain control of your life.

✎ What does Lamentations 3:22-23 mean to you as you seek God's guidance?

Grace is just as free today as it was yesterday. Each day offers a new supply. God will never fail you because He loves you so much.

 Thank You, Father God, for Your faithfulness in loving me and giving me Your grace every day of my life.

Heavenly Father, I seek Your guidance in living a life to fulfill the great expectations You have for me.

DAY 4: *Serve God with the Right Motive*

Elizabeth spent many years of her life working with disadvantaged young people. Admirers commended her for her work, but Elizabeth saw herself in a different light. She suffered from tremendous guilt because of wrong choices she made earlier in her life. She believed doing enough good deeds would improve her standing with God.

Elizabeth was doing the right thing with the wrong motive. Our motive for service to God should stem from an overflow of love and gratitude for who He is and what He has done for us.

✎ What does Colossians 1:10 say is the purpose of good works?

✎ According to Ephesians 2:9, why did God not choose to save you by good works?

≫ Isaiah 64:6 gives another reason our righteous acts will not save us. What is it?

Your boasting would take away God's glory and bring glory to yourself. The result would be arrogance and pride. You can never be good enough to merit God's grace! Do not try to use good deeds to cover up some basic weakness, past pain or wrong choices that break fellowship with God. Just as good works will not bring salvation, neither will they produce a healthy lifestyle. To develop a healthy lifestyle, good habits have to be developed. Keeping your Commitment Record is one helpful habit in reaching your goal for First Place. This daily record guides you in the nutrition your body needs and helps you with fulfilling the other commitments of prayer, Bible study, Scripture memory, exercise and encouragement. Use it daily, and it will help you make wise choices throughout the day.

≫ What other things can you do to help you live a healthier lifestyle?

The role of good works is to honor God and testify to the living faith that is in you. The Christian walk will naturally lead to Christlike deeds. When others see Christ in you as you minister and serve Him, they will be drawn to Him.

Heavenly Father, I seek Your help in overcoming my attitudes toward the works I do in Your name. Let them always be for Your glory and honor and because of my overwhelming desire to serve You.

Father God, I thank You for every opportunity You give me to serve You and bring glory to Your name.

DAY 5: *Rely on God*

The world may tell you that you are worthless; God's truth says you are His creation. The world insists that others' approval is most important; God's truth is that His acceptance of you is all that matters. The world tells you that you are hopeless and cannot change; God's truth tells you not to rely on willpower but on God's power to make changes in your life.

➤ According to Colossians 1:11-14 (and especially verse 11), what are two qualities you possess through God's power?

➤ Complete the following statements using verses 12 and 13:

He has qualified you to share in the_____of the

_____.

He rescued you from the _____ of

_____ and brought you into the

_____ of _____.

Everyone could use a little more endurance when the going gets tough, and who among you could not do with more patience. These qualities come from relying on God. You are qualified to share in the inheritance of the saints of the kingdom of light. Your life can be totally different when you rely completely on God in all circumstances.

➤ What are we to do even in difficult times, according to Philippians 4:6?

➤ What is the promise in verse 7 (if we do as instructed in v. 6)?

➤ In what practical ways would your life be different if you relied on God's power to achieve your First Place goals?

Show God your appreciation for your First Place group by letting your leaders know how much they encourage you and by encouraging a fellow group member with a phone call, a card or a message in person.

 Heavenly Father, I give thanks to You for providing a group like First Place to encourage me in reaching my goals for a healthier lifestyle.

Dear Lord, help me today to fully rely on You and let Your peace guard my mind and heart.

DAY 6: *Reflections*

You may be familiar with the hymn "Amazing Grace." It is the basis for the title and topic of this week's study. After 2,000 years, God's grace is still amazing. God loved you so much that He was willing for Jesus to die for your sins so you could inherit the eternal life He planned for you. He makes you to be holy and blameless through the blood of Jesus Christ.

You can believe God's promises without any doubts. He is the One by whom and for whom all things were made (see John 1:3). You can accept His gifts to you as His child. He gives those gifts freely. You could not and cannot earn them. Nothing qualifies you for the gift of salvation. All you have to do is accept God's grace for you, a sinner set free. Review this week's memory verse, and believe the promise.

God's Word is His book of promises for you to use in your life every day. You can fully rely on Him to supply all your needs.

Take time to write the memory verse in your prayer journal. As you read passages from the Bible for your daily study, write down verses you particularly like or that have special meaning for you. Think about verses you may have already memorized in the past. Reinforce those verses. Look them up and repeat them. You may find you have a great bank of Scriptures that you have deposited over the years.

Thank You, Father God, for making me a part of Your chosen people, a royal priesthood, a holy nation, a people who belong to You that I may declare the praises of You who called me out of darkness into Your wonderful light (see 1 Peter 2:9).

Lord God, put Your words in my mouth and cover me with the shadow of Your hand. You set the heavens in place and laid the foundations of the earth. You say to Your children, "You are my people" (see Isaiah 51:16).

DAY 7: *Reflections*

Besides having memorized verses ready to encourage you in times of difficulty another reason for memorizing Scripture is to help you overcome temptation and your enemy, Satan, who prowls around like a roaring lion looking for someone to devour (see 1 Peter 5:8). If you use God's Word in times of temptation as Jesus did, you will defeat your enemy.

A stronghold in your life can create a barrier between you and God, and it will give Satan an advantage as he attacks you at your weakest point. What is a stronghold? God's Word describes it as anything that sets itself against the knowledge of God (see 2 Corinthians 10:5). Anything in your life can become a stronghold from your eating and health habits to depression, stress, guilt, low self-esteem or pride. Remember, if anything gets in the way of your relationship with God, it can become a stronghold.

When you are secure in God's Word, God's love and God's will, Satan must flee from you. God gives you the weapons you need. They are weapons with divine power to demolish strongholds (see 2 Corinthians 10:4). Satan loses all power when confronted by the weapons of God's Word and prayer.

Memorizing Scripture gives you a strength and ability to meet every temptation. It is an important part of putting on the full armor of God (see Ephesians 6:10-18). Personalize verses by putting your name in key places and restating them in your own words. This will give you ownership of the verses and will help you apply them to your life.

Use the following verse prayers taken from *Praying God's Word* as you strive to overcome temptations and break down strongholds:

Some trust in chariots and some in horses, but I trust in the name of You, the Lord my God. My enemy will be brought to his knees and ultimately fall, but I will rise up and stand firm (see Psalm 20:7-8).[1]

Father God, I thank You because I am in Christ; Satan, the prince of this world, has no hold on me (see John 14:30).[2]

Father, I know I have been saved, through faith—and this not from myself, it is a gift You have given me—not by works, so that I cannot boast (see Ephesians 2:8-9).

Notes
1. Beth Moore, *Praying God's Word* (Nashville, TN: Broadman and Holman, 2000), p. 317.
2. Ibid., p. 326.

GROUP PRAYER REQUESTS   TODAY'S DATE:_____

NAME	REQUEST	RESULTS

THE POSITIVE
POWER OF PEACE

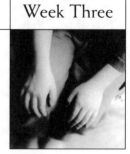

MEMORY VERSE
He himself is our peace, who has made the two one
and has destroyed the barrier, the dividing
wall of hostility, by abolishing in his flesh the
law with its commandments and regulations.
Ephesians 2:14-15

Two neighbors involved in a property dispute had a lawyer draw up an agreement. The neighbors signed the document, but the breach between them continued. A respected friend of both parties brought the two together in an attempt to achieve harmony. Because their common friend chose to be a peacemaker, these two finally settled their disagreement.

Christ is the ultimate model of a peacemaker. His peace draws people together, breaking down stereotypes and uniting them in love for each other. In this week's study, you will explore how to gain peace within yourself and peace with others.

DAY 1: *Christ Is Peace*

Christ's peace is an essential part of the precious inheritance you have in Him.

›› Reread the memory verse, Ephesians 2:14-15. How is Christ our peace?

Paul drew a parallel between what Christ did for us on the cross and the dividing walls that existed in the Temple of His day. In the Temple, Gentiles could only enter the first court. A wall kept them away from other temple areas, and a tablet announced that instant death awaited any Gentile who proceeded past the wall. That wall effectively shut out the Gentiles from the presence of God.

⇥ What dividing walls keep you from experiencing the presence of God?

⇥ In Jude 20-21, what three things does Jude urge Christians to do in faith for themselves?

⇥ According to verses 22-23, what are you to do for others?

These acts toward others will bring down the dividing walls in your life. Christ loved all men and women and offers the same love, mercy and grace to every one of us. Because of Calvary, God has forgiven you. Christ's blood paid for your peace.

⇥ According to Philippians 4:6-9, what must you do to have the peace of God?

Practicing the principles you have been taught and have received from God will bring you the peace that only the God of peace can give.

 Thank You, Heavenly Father, for Your promise of peace when we are obedient and seek Your guidance and will.

Lord, may the peace that surpasses all understanding be in my heart and soul today.

DAY 2: *His Law Brings Peace*

People who work in the area of criminal justice are referred to as peace officers. They bring individuals and communities peace by enforcing the law.

⇢ Consider Ephesians 2:15; what did Paul mean when he wrote that Christ abolished the law?

Jesus came to tell people that they could never earn God's approval by keeping Jewish ceremonial law. In the first place, the average person was unable to know, let alone keep, the bulky, man-made laws of the Jewish Talmud. Even the Pharisees spent a lifetime discussing and interpreting the law, and they were guilty of striving to keep the letter of the law while missing the purpose behind it.

⇢ Although the Pharisees were teaching the law, what did they forget, according to Jesus in Matthew 23:23-26?

⇢ What does Romans 7:7 say is the purpose of God's law?

⇢ What seems to be the contradiction between Jesus' words in Matthew 5:17 and Paul's teaching in Ephesians 2:15 about Jesus' purpose?

⇢ How can we reconcile these two seemingly contradictory statements?

➤ Read Galatians 2:16 and 5:4-6. Since keeping the law does not justify us, what does?

God gave us the law so that we would know right from wrong. God knew that because of your sin nature you would never be righteous on your own merit to save yourself from the penalty for sin (see Romans 6:23). Through faith, you accept Jesus' payment for your sins on the cross. It is Christ's righteousness alone that gives you access to God.

Perhaps you feel God is displeased with you over health and lifestyle choices. You may experience this feeling as a barrier between yourself and God. However, there is no stronghold that cannot be broken down through God's Word.

Confess your barriers or strongholds and accept His free gift of salvation. Focus on your faith in Him as you live for Him today.

 Father, thank You for the free gift of salvation through the price Your Son paid at Calvary.

Holy Lord, help me to bring down any barrier I erect that sets itself against You. Fill me with power through Your Word to demolish my strongholds.

DAY 3: *He Gives Peace*

A well-known commercial describes a certain product as "the gift that keeps on giving." In John 14:27, Jesus said, "Peace I leave with you; my peace I give to you." God's peace didn't end with the death and resurrection of His Son. It is a gift that keeps on giving.

➤ Match the statements describing God's peace to their correct Scripture reference.

_____ God's peace is a by-product of the   a. Philippians 4:7
Holy Spirit in you.

_____ God's peace is a by-product   b.   Psalm 119:165
of obedience.

_____ God's peace is a by-product of faith,   c.   Galatians 5:22
not understanding.

If Jesus is your source of peace, the by-products of His peace are benefits you will experience in your daily life. His peace cannot be explained by the human mind, and it guards the hearts and minds of those who live His Word and obey His commands. Peace is also one of the ways the Holy Spirit demonstrates His presence in your life.

➤ What is Jesus' promise of peace in John 14:27?

Martha sat in the emergency room waiting area. Her son paced the floor in front of her with worry etched on his face. Finally he turned to her and asked, "How can you sit there so calm with Dad back there maybe dying from his heart attack? Aren't you worried or afraid?" She smiled and answered, "I turned your Dad over to God. He's taking care of him right now. I don't have to worry or be afraid because God gave me His peace. Dad will be okay."

You can experience the peace that only God can give. He promised it to you as a gift of His inheritance, and God keeps His promises.

➤ How does the peace that God gives as part of your inheritance impact how you keep your First Place commitments? Check all that apply.

☐ I claim His peace when I am feeling stressed and out of control.

☐ I give my anxieties to Him instead of trying to cope with my fears.

☐ I am obedient to His command that I regard my body as His temple.

☐ I take the necessary steps to be at peace with myself, realizing that I may need to make changes in my lifestyle.

Share your commitment for peace with a fellow First Place group member. Ask that member to pray with you, and then pray for that person. God will help each of you to keep your commitments.

 Lord Jesus, thank You for giving me a peace that takes away my worry and fear.

Father God, grant me the power to keep the commitments I make to You. Fill me with Your Holy Spirit and grant me a willing spirit to sustain me.

DAY 4: *He Makes Peace*

Paul categorized Christ's work of ending separation as creating "one new man out of the two" (Ephesians 2:15). He overcame all that separates people from Christ and from one another. Christ opens the door to God for all people, whatever their backgrounds. Review Ephesians 2:14-16.

➤ Describe some characteristics you believe are true for a person reconciled to him- or herself, God and others.

Do you ever feel separated from God and/or other people? Are you overly critical of yourself or others? When you fail to meet a daily or weekly goal, do you feel you have disappointed God or those who care about you? Or do your shortcomings cause you to feel uncomfortable around other Christians?

➤ What question from the previous list might describe your feelings?

Christ will give you the power to overcome any obstacle that you believe you have. His forgiveness makes you whole.

➤ According to Romans 8:1-2, from what does Christ Jesus free you?

If Christ does not condemn you, you have no reason to condemn yourself or to allow anything to separate you from God and others.

➤ Describe one step you will take to set aside any condemnation you feel.

 Lord, I pray for Your guidance as You help me to take the step I listed here.

Father God, I thank You for setting me free from the law of sin and death and for the promise that there is no condemnation for me because of what Christ Jesus did.

DAY 5: *He Preaches Peace*

Besides representing peace and making peace, Jesus also preaches peace. He launched a mission of preaching peace to those who were far away and near (see Ephesians 2:17). The "near" persons probably referred to the Jews, and the "far away" meant the Gentiles. Or Paul may have been referring to the overall task of proclaiming the gospel worldwide.

➤ According to Ephesians 2:17-18, to whom do we have access as a result of Christ's preaching?

Circle the number that best describes where you are in relation to feeling Christ's peace.

1	2	3	4	5
Far away				Near

⇒ What would it take for you to feel nearer to Christ's peace?

Many people attempt to find contentment in a lifestyle that glorifies overindulgence and pleasure. Others lead rushed, stressful lifestyles that don't include time for keeping the body, mind or spirit fit. Instead of lasting peace, they feel despair. Only by giving Christ first place can you achieve true peace. Seek Him first. He will make His ways known to you, including ways you can care for your body, His temple.

⇒ What three things does Paul tell the believers to do in Hebrews 10:22-25?

⇒ According to verses 19-21, why can we do those things listed in the previous question?

If you feel Christ's peace, think of someone in your group, church or other realm of influence with whom you can share His peace. If you need Christ's peace, tell Him your needs and commit to drawing nearer to Him.

 Heavenly Father, I seek the peace You promise in Your Word, for I know it will guard my heart and mind against my enemy.

Lord, because You have been so merciful to me, I want to share Your love and peace with those who may not know You. Let my life be a testimony of Your love and peace.

DAY 6: *Reflections*

In this week's study we learned about the peace that comes from knowing God. God's peace is a positive influence and power in your life. You can know God's peace through your knowledge of Jesus Christ. God's peace is a gift of your inheritance and is one that keeps on giving. His peace destroys barriers and walls of hostility as you rest in the saving grace of the Lord Jesus Christ.

Mark 4:35-41 tells about the disciples being afraid and waking Jesus when a sudden storm threatened to capsize their boat. Jesus calmed the waves and the sea with three words: "Quiet! Be still!" (v. 39). His words will calm the raging storms in your life. His words will give you peace. Christ Himself is the peace that "transcends all understanding" (Philippians 4:7).

Claim God's peace as your peace. Let Him calm the waves causing stress in your life. Walk with Him, read His Word and study the Scriptures, and you will find the peace God so freely offers you as His child.

 Lord God, I know You will rescue me from every evil attack and will bring me safely to Your heavenly kingdom. To You be glory for ever and ever (see 2 Timothy 4:18).

Thank You, Heavenly Father, for the grace that brings salvation to me and that has appeared to all men (see Titus 2:11).

Father God, Your divine power has given me everything I need for life and godliness through my knowledge of You who called me by Your own glory and goodness (see 2 Peter 1:3).

DAY 7: *Reflections*

Today we discover the third purpose in memorizing Scripture. Having God's Word in your heart gives you guidance that will direct your decisions and activities throughout your day. His Word will be a lamp to your feet and a light for your path (see Psalm 119:105).

Beginning each day with a quiet time of reading, studying and memorizing God's Word brings you to the throne of grace and into a closer, more intimate relationship with God. This time with God equips you for the day ahead and everything Satan tries to throw in your way. God will lead you and give you guidance for the day ahead as you commune with Him.

You are memorizing one Scripture a week as part of your commitment to First Place. Expand that habit and begin looking for Scriptures that will help you to grow in the knowledge of Jesus Christ. A good Bible concordance will help you to find verses and topics of particular interest to you. Ask God to help you recall verses as you pray each day. Using God's Word in prayer gives your prayers extra power and strength as you strive to bring down the strongholds that threaten to undermine your relationship with Him.

You now have three excellent purposes for memorizing Scripture. Remember to use the Scripture Memory Music CD and *Walking in the Word* book in your endeavor to learn more of God's Word.

The following prayers use Scriptures to tell of God's guidance for your life:

 Lord God, show me Your ways and teach me Your paths; guide me in Your truth and teach me, for You are God, my Savior, and my hope is in You all day long (see Psalm 25:4-5).

O Lord, I am always with You; You hold me by my right hand. You guide me with Your counsel, and afterward You will take me into Your glory (see Psalm 73:23-24).

Heavenly Father, You promised to guide me always; You will satisfy my needs in a sun-scorched land and will strengthen my frame so that I am like a well-watered garden (see Isaiah 58:11).

Thank You, Father, for sending the Spirit of truth; for when He comes, He will guide me into all truth (see John 16:7).

It is You, my peace, who has made the two one and has destroyed the barrier, the dividing wall of hostility, by abolishing in Your flesh the law with its commandments and regulations (see Ephesians 2:14-15).

Group Prayer Requests   Today's Date:_____

Name	Request	Results

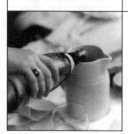
GOD'S
100 PERCENT

MEMORY VERSE

Know this love that surpasses knowledge—
that you may be filled to the measure
of all the fullness of God.

Ephesians 3:19

In the first two chapters of Ephesians, Paul described our inheritance as children of the heavenly Father. God offers His inheritance as a grace gift. Ephesians 3 clarifies what may seem to be a mystery. Through the inspiration of the Holy Spirit, Paul shared a truth God had waited until this age to disclose.

DAY 1: *No Barriers*

Do you enjoy reading a mystery? Many people like solving puzzles and playing the role of amateur detective. Let's discover the answer to a mystery.

➤ What is the truth that had not been revealed until the present age, according to Ephesians 3:4-6?

Although Paul was describing the racial implications of Gentiles becoming Christians, the truth for us is that because of Calvary all people come to Jesus on an equal basis. Until the coming of Christ, Israel was the one nation through which God had spoken. Israel's role was to show other nations the one true God. However, God's plan has always been to extend His love to all nations, races and cultures.

➤ To whom does the "whosoever" refer in John 3:16 (*KJV*)?

➤ Can you fully accept the fact that God loves all people completely?

   ☐ Yes   ☐ No

➤ If you answered no, what barriers are in the way of your accepting this truth?

➤ What is the promise found in Romans 8:35-39?

➤ Do you know that there is absolutely nothing you can do to make God stop loving you?

   ☐ Yes   ☐ No

Sometimes things happen in life that may cause you to feel unloved, even by God.

➤ What may have happened to make you feel unloved by God?

Struggles with weight or other health issues may cause you to feel that you are less acceptable to others. You may also feel less loved by God than those who do not appear to face these challenges. Do not despair. Read the verses in Romans 8 again. You can believe God's Word. Once you accept God's love and allow the Holy Spirit to reign in your life, nothing will be able to separate you from the love of God in Christ Jesus.

Heavenly Father, fill me anew with the awareness that I am Your precious child, fully loved and accepted by You.

Thank You, dear Lord, for the promise that nothing will separate me from Your love.

DAY 2: *Unsurpassing Knowledge*

A young child was busily drawing a picture. His mother asked him what he was drawing. "A picture of God," he announced. His mother explained that no one knows what God looks like. He replied, "They will when I am through."

➤ According to Ephesians 3:19, to what measure will God's love fill you?

➤ According to Psalms 44:21 and 94:11, how well does God know you?

Paul says that no one knows the depths of Christ's love, yet the psalmist tells you God knows you completely!

➤ How is it possible to be fully known and fully loved?

➤ Write a prayer thanking God for His love, even when you are feeling or being unlovable.

Paul encouraged the Ephesians to make every effort to know God's love—the love which he had just said is beyond knowing! In Christ, Christians can know the unknowable. Like the child with the drawing, Paul in essence is saying, "When Christ gets through with you, you will know His unknowable love."

Paul's ultimate goal was that Christians might be filled with the fullness of God. The fullness of God means all God wants for you, God's best—His 100 percent.

➤ In each of the following areas, write the changes you need to make to receive God's best:

🍎 My relationship with the Father

🍎 Care of my body

🍎 A balanced lifestyle

Heavenly Father, help me to know Your unlimited love and remove any barriers that may keep me from feeling worthy of that love.

Father God, I praise Your name for loving me with such a great love that is as high as the heavens above the earth and deeper than the deepest sea.

DAY 3: *Life to the Fullest*

A child once asked an older relative if she were a Christian. "Parts of me are," came the reply. The woman was afraid that total commitment to Christ would deprive her of certain things or behaviors which she did not want to give up.

➤ How would the belief that living the Christian life means depriving yourself of something affect your life?

➤ What have you given up in order to live the Christian life?

➤ In releasing your life to Christ, what have you gained?

➤ In John 10:7-10, to what did Jesus compare Himself?

➤ What kind of life did Jesus promise believers?

Christ came so that you could have abundant life "filled to the measure of all the fullness of God" (Ephesians 3:19). Do you view the Christian life as a process of adding to your life in abundance or a life of deprivation?

In what ways can you attest to the fact that you have abundant life because of Christ's power in you? Check all that apply.

☐ Courage to face difficulties
☐ Awareness of His presence when I pray
☐ Ability to resist temptation
☐ Companionship when I am lonely
☐ Guidance in times of indecision
☐ Other _____

"Filled to the measure of all the fullness of God" means there is no shortage of ways He wants to bless you. Will you let Him?

Thank You, Father, for loving me and giving me the blessings of my life. May I always be grateful and bless Your precious name.

Lord, I pray for Your continuous blessings on me as You fill my cup to overflowing each day.

DAY 4: *His Place in Your Life*

When you received salvation, you became heir to everything that is God's and everything *is* His. When His Holy Spirit came to dwell in you, He did not come to merely inhabit your soul, but also your emotions, mind and body. This habitation includes every area of life that causes you to stumble or be separated from God in any way.

➤ Have you ever believed that you somehow had less of God in you than you did when you were saved? If so, describe the situation.

Life's circumstances may make you feel as if you have less of God dwelling in you. Disappointments, mistakes and injustices may cause you to feel removed from God. You may carry around a load of shame or grief because of others' or your own mistakes, but God hasn't removed Himself from your difficulties. Nothing can remove God's presence from you.

➤ What is the assurance of God's presence found in Psalm 139:7-12?

Once you become a child of God, no matter where you go or what you do, He will be with you. No matter what you experience, God is with you. What a wonderful promise! Although you may feel God is far away when you are in pain or doubt, He is only a prayer away.

Only those who have never asked Jesus to be Savior and Lord of their lives are cut off from God's intimate fellowship and denied the blessing of His inheritance. If this describes you, take this opportunity to accept God's invitation to salvation. Speak with your First Place leader about this important decision. He or she will pray with you.

If you make such a decision and pray for God's forgiveness, sign your name and write the date after reading the following statement:

> On this day I choose to honor God with my life and body. I accept Christ as my personal Savior.

Signed:_____

Date: _____

➣ After reading 1 John 5:12-13, explain how you can know you have eternal life in Christ.

➣ Write the promise found in 2 Corinthians 5:17-18.

Ask God for His power to enable you to live as one who has been bought with a costly price—Christ's death—that you might be free to walk in new paths.

Thank You, Father God, for making me a new creation in Christ. Help me to live out that truth in my daily life.

Heavenly Father, I pray for Your wisdom, power and strength in my daily life to lead me into new paths of service for You.

DAY 5: *His Power*

You may have heard the question: "If you do not feel as close to God as you once did, who moved?" If you desire to move closer to God, examine the nine commitments to First Place. They are designed to help you have a more intimate relationship with God.

➤ List the commitment that you need to work on because it will be most helpful in your spiritual life.

➤ According to Ephesians 3:16, whose power will enable you to keep the commitments you listed?

Paul knew the secret of living a life with the power of God. He found himself in many circumstances that placed him in danger. Officials imprisoned him and caused him to suffer. He had very little in the way of material possessions. Despite his hardships, Paul knew the source of power and strength for victory over sin and death.

➤ According to Philippians 4:12-13, what was Paul's secret?

➤ What is the promise in Philippians 4:19?

You have this same promise. Rely on His power, and He will supply everything you need to have a closer relationship with Him.

Relying on your own strength may bring some success for some amount of time. God's strength and power enable you to win daily victories for all of life! Allow God to make you aware of His strength already in you. Ask Him to give you the confidence that you can achieve your goals and be successful through Him who gives you strength and supplies all your needs.

Heavenly Father, thank You for Your promise to supply all my needs through Your precious Son, Jesus Christ.

Lord God, I ask You to help me learn to be content in every situation I may encounter in my daily living.

DAY 6: *Reflections*

This week's memory verse declares a love that surpasses knowledge so that you may be filled with the measure of the fullness of God. God offers His grace to you freely as part of your inheritance as a child of God. You know of God's love and His mercy toward you as a sinner, but so much about God seems unknowable.

When you commit yourself wholly to God, He will fill you with His love and, ultimately, you will know what God wants for your life. He wants you to live your life to the fullest through Him. Joining First Place was a step in the direction of seeking the best God has to offer for your life. He loves you when you feel unloved. He is with you when you feel alone, and He cares for you in any and every situation. When you seek God first, everything else you need will be given to you (see Matthew 6:33).

When disappointments come and you don't reach the goals you set in First Place, you may feel you have failed. This is not true. You simply haven't finished your journey toward being the best you can be. Don't give up. Instead, get up and continue on your journey. Be sure that Satan will tempt you to give up many times along your journey. You may have setbacks and detours, but if you persevere, you can reach your destination.

Remember to pray daily to ask God to lead you and to give you the strength you need to be successful one day at a time.

Heavenly Father, my prayer is that my love for You may abound more and more in knowledge and insight so that I may discern what is best and be pure and blameless until Your return (see Philippians 1:9-10).

Although I may stumble, Father God, I will not fall because You uphold me with Your hand (see Psalm 37:24).

For I have not received a spirit that makes me a slave to fear, but I have received the Spirit of sonship and by that I cry out to You, Abba, Father (see Romans 8:15).

In You, O Lord, my heart rejoices, for I trust in Your holy name (see Psalm 33:21).

DAY 7: *Reflections*

The fourth purpose for memorizing Scripture is that it gives you a valuable tool to use as you witness to others about what God has done in your life. You may already be familiar with Scriptures that can help you lead someone to the saving knowledge of Jesus Christ. The book of Romans has many verses that are a great help in witnessing.

Many times when the opportunity for witnessing arises, you may not have your Bible with you. Think about how confident you can be when you have the words of God written in your heart and mind.

At some point in your Christian walk, you may be asked to give your testimony as to how God has worked in your life. That testimony is made even more powerful as people listen to God's Word coming from your heart. Find Bible verses that express your own personal testimony. Memorize them and use them when you tell others about Jesus Christ and His great love for you.

God's Word is one of the treasures of your inheritance. It is to be used every day, not put away in a safety deposit box for some future date. Like fine silver, the Word of God will grow more lustrous with daily use. Dip into the treasure box, and claim the blessings God promises you through His Word.

If you're still shaky about memorizing Scripture, memorize the verse one phrase at a time. Dividing the verse into components that are meaningful to you, will make the process of memorization easier. Work with it until you are able to quote the verse word perfect. Don't expect it to happen the first time or two that you say the verse. Give it time and keep at it. You might even ask your leader to help you with your verses each week.

If you find Scripture memorization to be easy for you, check with others in your group who may be having trouble and offer to help them.

Use the resources and tools available from First Place, and ask your heavenly Father to help you. You have too many resources at your disposal to say "I can't do it." You just might not have found the right method for you as yet.

The following are verses you can use in your witness to others:

Father God, thank You for Your gift of salvation because I know that all have sinned and come short of Your glory (see Romans 3:23).

Heavenly Father, thank You for demonstrating Your love for me in that while I was still a sinner, Christ died for me (see Romans 5:8).

Holy God, I confess with my mouth that Jesus is Lord and I believe in my heart that You, O God, raised Him from the dead and because of this I am redeemed (see Romans 10:9).

O Lord, help me to flee from sin and to pursue righteousness, godliness, faith, love, endurance and gentleness (see 1 Timothy 6:11).

Father God, I know the love that surpasses knowledge and am filled to the measure of all Your fullness (see Ephesians 3:19).

Group Prayer Requests Today's Date:_____

Name	Request	Results

MATURITY: A CHOICE

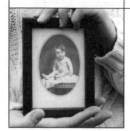

MEMORY VERSE

You were taught, with regard to your former way of life, to put off your old self . . . and to put on the new self, created to be like God in true righteousness and holiness.

Ephesians 4:22-24

Babies become children who grow into teenagers and then into adults. A two-year-old child cannot suddenly decide, "I will remain 30 inches tall and weigh 30 pounds." Physical growth is not an option for a healthy infant. When a child is properly nourished and in good health, he or she will grow—there is no way to stop it.

However, spiritual maturity is not an automatic process; it takes work and discipline. In this week's study look for ways God shows you how to grow up in Christ.

DAY 1: *Becoming a New Creation*

When you become a Christian, your old, sinful self is discarded. Much like a caterpillar shedding its cocoon, you emerge as a new creature. Did you ever wonder if the emerging new butterfly needs time to adjust to the ability to fly? Does it ever long for predictable days on the ground or in the cocoon? Are you sometimes tempted to revert to your old life as an unbeliever with its comfortable ruts?

➤ Consider 1 Corinthians 1:18; what are some aspects of the Christian life that might seem foolish to non-Christians?

⟫ According to 1 Corinthians 2:14, why can't the non-Christian accept spiritual things?

People who are not spiritually minded may laugh at Christians and their foolishness. Those without Christ wear spiritual blinders and can't understand the Christian's interest in church activities, prayer and Bible study. Our faith in an unseen God is foreign to them. Their natural inclination is to reject the things of Christ.

⟫ Can you remember when you were without Christ? Describe some of the things that seemed important before you accepted Christ but are no longer important now.

⟫ What are some things that have become more important to you now that you are a Christian?

The natural person is centered in him- or herself and is unprotected from Satan's temptation. Christians must be self-controlled and alert because their enemy, Satan, "walks around like a roaring lion seeking someone to devour" (1 Peter 5:8). Whenever you let down your guard and think you can take care of yourself through willpower and self-discipline, Satan will jump in and take advantage.

⟫ Have you ever thought you could have better health and fitness by merely being strong willed and self-disciplined? Describe what happened.

Only God's power—not willpower—can help you be strong in the face of temptation. When unbelievers scoff at you for believing in the foolishness of the Cross, remind yourself that you are a new creation.

➻ List some ways in which you can grow in Christ in the coming weeks.

Thank You, Heavenly Father, for creating a new me when I became a Christian and for giving me the Holy Spirit to guide and lead me.

Father God, help me to grow and mature and become closer to You through this First Place program and through reading and studying Your Word.

DAY 2: *Being Governed by the Flesh*

Paul, in his letter to the Romans, gave us some good news and some bad news. The good news is that you have a new nature because of the indwelling Christ. The bad news is that you still have the old nature trying to take over. These two natures war against each other.

➻ What is at the heart of the problem that Paul described in Romans 7:21-25?

➻ Is there a part of your own sinful nature that sometimes wants to take control? Describe what happens.

➤ What are the two types of Christians identified in 1 Corinthians 3:1-3?

Spiritual Christians are mature in their faith because they can eat solid food—those things that take some work to chew and digest. Worldly Christians survive on milk—those things that are easy to swallow.

➤ What are examples of immaturity in worldly Christians?

Worldly Christians are saved but don't act much different from their unsaved friends. They allow jealousy to cause competition among them. Their salvation is secure; but like the unbelieving world, they are governed by the flesh. Worldly Christians are dissatisfied and unfulfilled because they don't follow the will of God. A place is reserved for them in heaven with Christ, but they will miss the riches He planned for them on this earth.

➤ Do you sometimes live as though Christ had not given you a new nature?

☐ Yes   ☐ No

➤ Check the behaviors common to a worldly Christian that you don't want in your life.

☐ Envy and greed   ☐ Arguments and quarrels with others
☐ Impure thoughts   ☐ Selfish attitude

A Christian who wants an intimate relationship with God wouldn't want anything in his or her life that would create a barrier against that relationship. In the pursuit of spiritual things, do you sometimes neglect your physical growth and live as someone who doesn't care about health and fitness? Christ will give you the ability to set aside that nature and take on traits to help you be in better health. His power can give you the strength to take proper care of your body, mind and soul.

Thank You, Father God, for my First Place group. Bless each of us as we set aside our sinful natures and think about the Christlike traits we want to develop.

Father, I pray Your blessings on me as I put aside my old nature and live as a new creature fully committed to serving You.

DAY 3: *Giving Christ Control*

Today you will learn more about giving Christ control.

Mature believers leave behind the things of the old nature that are contrary to what God wants for their lives, and they choose to walk in the path of the Spirit daily.

➤ Write Galatians 2:20 and personalize it by inserting your name after every use of the word "I."

➤ How are you to live a spiritual life?

➤ According to Ephesians 4:1-7, how are we to live?

➤ What is the wonderful news in verse 7?

A spiritual Christian sets aside old ways as though he or she has buried them. Some of those old ways may include improper health habits in diet and exercise. As one who desires maturity in Christ, offer each part of yourself in sweet surrender to Him. God's transforming power can conquer the old nature and replace it with a new, divine one.

➤ After reading Ephesians 3:20-21, write the verses in your own words as a prayer.

Heavenly Father, I acknowledge You as Lord over every part of my life. Help me to live my life according to Your will.

Lord God, I pray for You to take control of my life and help me to overcome the temptations that threaten to draw me away from You.

DAY 4: *Taking the Mind Captive*

Each of the three types of persons described in this study—the natural person, the worldly Christian, the spiritual Christian—have made choices. The natural person chooses to reject the things of Christ. The worldly Christian picks and chooses among the things of Christ. The spiritual person seeks to accept all of Christ.

Choosing to be a spiritual Christian requires discipline to leave behind anything that distracts you from God's eternal path for your life. What you receive instead—God's delight in you and your fellowship with Him—will be more pleasing and satisfying than any substitute could ever be.

You may say, "This really sounds great, but practically speaking, how do I go about setting aside things in my life that differ from God's plan for me?" Since actions spring from thoughts, you must begin by gaining control of your mind.

➵ According to 2 Corinthians 10:3-5, what did Paul urge Christians to do?

➵ What aspects of your life might be in opposition to God's plan for you?

Every Christian needs to overcome certain temptations, whether they be food choices, actions or attitudes.

➵ What is one temptation that you would like to gain control over?

➵ What actions could you take to demolish the thoughts or actions for this particular temptation?

Changing deeply ingrained thoughts and actions, whether food related or not, takes time. Don't be discouraged if you don't improve instantly or are drawn back into the temptation and give in. When you ask the Lord to renew your mind—as the memory verse affirms—results will follow.

Heavenly Father, I pray that You will help me set aside all thoughts or actions that are contrary to Your will.

Lord God, fill me with Your divine power to demolish the strongholds in my life.

DAY 5: *Activating Christ's Mind in You*

Have you ever been challenged *not* to think of a pink elephant? Telling yourself not to think certain thoughts does not solve your problem in trying to get your mind under control. You must replace negative/wrong thoughts with positive/righteous ones.

⟫ According to Philippians 4:8, on what should we think?

⟫ According to Colossians 3:1-2, where should your thoughts be directed?

⟫ Name three negative/wrong thoughts that plague you, and next to them write positive/righteous thoughts with which you could replace them.

Negative/Wrong	Positive/Righteous

➤ Match the following statements with their corresponding Scripture references:

_____ Meditate on God's love.   a. Psalm 1:2

_____ Meditate on God's Word.   b. Psalm 48:9

_____ Set your mind on what the   c. Romans 8:5-6
Holy Spirit desires.

Occupy your mind with Christ-honoring thoughts. Replace the thoughts that lead to wrong actions as soon as you become aware of them. One way to mature in Christ is to ask others to pray with you about specific character traits that you want to develop. If you do not feel comfortable praying with a First Place group member, then call or meet with a friend and share your prayer request.

Heavenly Father, help me to keep my thoughts on things above and let me meditate on Your Word daily.

Lord, thank You for giving me the opportunity to serve You and to search Your Word for comfort and guidance.

DAY 6: *Reflections*

This week's memory verse instructs us to put off our old self and our former way of life. When you become a Christian, you are created anew to be like Jesus in righteousness and holiness.

Our ideal is the perfect life of Jesus Christ. Although we can never reach the perfection of Jesus, we can take on many of the qualities He demonstrated during His ministry. We can love, minister, witness, comfort and serve just as He did. He has given us an instruction book, the Bible, to show us how to live the lives He wants us to have.

You have the choice of living in fullness with Him or living your own way and missing the blessings He has set aside just for you. Remember, spiritual maturity doesn't come overnight. You must develop it over your lifetime of service to Him. Whether you became a Christian as a young child or as a full-grown adult, you must continue to grow in the Lord.

You can restart that journey today if you have strayed off the path. You can continue on the path you began as a new creation in Him.

Keeping the First Place commitments will help you stay on track as you journey toward Christian maturity. Bible study, Scripture memory, prayer and reading God's Word, along with taking care of your physical body, all help in your efforts to put away your old self and pursue righteousness and holiness.

Lord God, cleanse me from all unrighteousness and make me an instrument for noble purpose, made holy, useful to You and prepared to do any good work (see 2 Timothy 2:21).

Thank You, Father, for not giving me a spirit of timidity but a spirit of power, of love and of self-discipline (see 2 Timothy 1:7).

Lord, help me to remember it is You who works in me to will and to act according to Your purpose (see Philippians 2:13).

DAY 7: *Reflections*

With the completion of this week's study, you are halfway through this session. By now you may be wondering if you'll make it to the end. Take heart and don't give up. Many times the last half is more rewarding than the first. This brings us to the fifth purpose for memorizing Scripture.

Memorizing Scripture gives us immediate access to all of God's promises when we need them. God sent promises to comfort, heal, forgive, give hope, guide our paths and bring us closer to Him. When God's promises are written on our hearts, we can be confident in His power to help us succeed in our endeavors to become more mature in Christ.

Another way to memorize Scripture is to practice saying it regularly. When you're driving in your car, waiting for an appointment or having your quiet time, repeat the verse several times. Review all the verses you have learned so far at least once a week to keep them fresh in your mind. Be on the lookout for new verses to add to your list.

Using God's Word in your prayers unleashes divine power. In *Praying God's Word*, Beth Moore teaches us how to take our thoughts and make them captive. That is done by choosing to think Christ's thoughts about any situation or stronghold instead of our own thoughts or those Satan might put in our minds. She states, "What are Christ's thoughts? The Word of God revealed to us."[1]

What promises are revealed to you through the Word of God? The following prayers are based on promises found in God's Word:

Father God, You have promised to wipe away all my tears. There will be no more death or mourning or crying or pain, for the old order of things will pass away. You have promised a new heaven and a new earth (see Revelation 21:1-4).

For You, Lord God, are gracious and merciful, and You will not turn Your face away from me if I return to You (see 2 Chronicles 30:9).

Lord, I claim Your promise for the plans You have for me. Your plans are to prosper me and not to harm me; plans to give me a hope and a future (see Jeremiah 29:11).

Father, I have been taught with regard to my former way of life to put off my old self and to put on my new self. I have been created to be like You in true righteousness and holiness; help me to live the life You have planned for me (see Ephesians 4:22-24).

Note
1. Beth Moore, *Praying God's Word* (Nashville, TN: Broadman and Holman, 2000), p. 7.

GROUP PRAYER REQUESTS   TODAY'S DATE:_____

NAME	REQUEST	RESULTS

A LOVE RELATIONSHIP

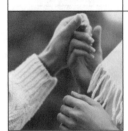

MEMORY VERSE

Live a life of love, just as Christ loved us and gave himself up for us as a fragrant offering and sacrifice to God.

Ephesians 5:2

Rachel glanced one more time at her image in the full-length mirror and adjusted her bridal veil. Her wedding day! As a young single, she had scoffed at the idea of spending the rest of her life with one man. Now one lifetime seemed too short to spend with Alex. What had changed Rachel's perspective? Their love relationship.

Before you became a Christian, spending an eternity with God may have seemed uninviting—even boring. Hopefully, now you are eagerly anticipating being with your Beloved Lord in heaven. The difference is the love relationship. In this week's study look for ways you can grow in your love for Him and for others.

DAY 1: *Imitate the Lord*

Jamie excitedly opened the package and found a bicycle reflector. She took the reflector into a dark closet to see it glow. But, of course, it did not. A reflector can only reflect light since it has no light source of its own.

Jesus called His disciples the light of the world (see Matthew 5:14). Believers are reflections of the one, true Light—the Lord Jesus Christ.

After reading Ephesians 5:1, complete the following statement:

➳ We are to imitate _____ as dearly _____ children.

You can imitate Christ as you reflect His love. You understood God's love because it was modeled through Christ's example of love and sacrifice.

➤ How did Jesus describe His relationship with His Father, according to John 14:31?

➤ And how did Jesus demonstrate His love?

➤ According to John 14:23, what is the proof of our love for Jesus?

➤ How well do you imitate Christ's obedience in terms of the way you treat your body?

☐ Complete obedience
☐ Partial obedience
☐ Lack of obedience

As a First Place member, you can be a positive example for others when they see you treat your body as the holy temple of God. They will be drawn to the light you reflect.

➤ What does Matthew 5:16 tell you to do with the light God gives you?

You can be a light in the darkness to show others the way to the Light of the world—Jesus. Obey God and love Him so that your love will reflect His love and be a shining beacon in a world of darkness.

Heavenly Father, help me to be obedient when I am tempted to stray from my commitment to You and my commitments to First Place.

Lord God, help me to be a shining light to others as I reflect Your love and mercy in my life.

DAY 2: *Live a Life of Love*

Jesus lived in perfect obedience to God and perfect love for others. We are to imitate Jesus in our love for others.

➤ What does the memory verse say about a life characterized by love?

When you imitate Jesus and love people with a sacrificial love, you please God because He loves everyone unconditionally.

➤ List the characteristics from Ephesians 4:30 that grieve the Holy Spirit.

➤ List the characteristics that please the Holy Spirit (v. 32).

Forgiveness is a key ingredient in love. God forgave your sin because of the blood of Christ. His forgiveness of you is related to your forgiveness of others.

➤ What does Matthew 6:14-15 say about forgiveness?

For years Martha denied having a brother. He sat in a prison cell, having been convicted of selling drugs. He lived a degenerate life separated from God—a life that included emotional abuse to the family, drug addiction and homosexuality. Martha didn't want anyone to know that she, a Christian, could have such a brother. After many years but while still in prison, her brother accepted Christ as his Savior. Martha refused to believe it and continued to deny that he was her brother. One morning in her prayer time, she realized something was different in her own life. The joy had gone and a heaviness had settled in her heart. For several days she tried to pray, but she only felt isolation and separation from God. She read the passage from Matthew and fell to her knees in prayer. She had put a barrier between herself and God by refusing to forgive her brother whom God had forgiven. She prayed for God to forgive her; then she wrote a letter to her brother asking his forgiveness for the years she had denied him. Today they have a wonderful relationship not only because of their blood but also through the blood of the Lamb, Jesus Christ, who was slain for their sin.

Without forgiveness of others, you cannot experience God's forgiving love for yourself. You may have people in your own life whom you need to forgive.

➤ Put a check by any person with whom you need to seek forgiveness.

☐ Sibling   ☐ Friend

☐ Parent   ☐ Child

☐ Fellow church member   ☐ Neighbor

☐ Spouse   ☐ Church leader

☐ Coworker   ☐ Other _____

As God loved you and forgave you, so must you love and forgive others. Go to that person you checked as soon as possible and talk with him or her about your relationship. God will honor the act even if the other person doesn't respond in a positive way. Your obedience will be a fragrant offering and sacrifice to God.

Heavenly Father, give me the strength and will to forgive those who have hurt or displeased me. Help me to love and forgive just as You love and forgive me.

Holy Lord, keep the bitter root of unforgiveness from rising up and causing trouble in my life and marring my witness of You.

DAY 3: *Love as Christ Loved You*

We might say we love hamburgers, love to go fishing, love that new movie and love our parents. The Greeks use three words for love to distinguish among the different kinds. *Agape* is the highest form of love, the kind of love God has for you.

➤ What did Jesus say about love in John 15:9?

➤ How did Jesus prove His love, according to John 15:13?

What an amazing and powerful love Jesus bestowed on us. He proved it with His own life! If we had been righteous, God-honoring people, perhaps it would have made sense for Jesus to give His life for us. But He gave His life in spite of our unrighteousness.

➤ What is your response to this sacrificial love as described in Romans 5:7-8?

Read John 15:12,17 and 1 John 3:16-18. Describe specific ways you can show sacrificial love for

🍎 A family member

🍎 A group member

🍎 A neighbor

🍎 A coworker

🐦 What is the command about love found in 1 John 3:23?

Are you being obedient to God's command? You can show your love for others in many different ways. Some examples of ways to show love are offering a ride to church to someone with no transportation; standing up for someone being falsely accused; sitting with a sick friend to allow family members time to take care of business; offering to help relieve a load for someone at work; taking time to visit with those who are ill or shut in. These acts of love will require time and energy, and maybe even money or possessions. Yet, by doing these acts, you express your love for others. In your prayer time today, ask God to show you ways you can help others in your family, First Place group, or circle of friends or coworkers.

Heavenly Father, thank You for loving me, and help me to love others as You love me.

O Lord, show me ways to give my love to others as an expression of my own love for You.

DAY 4: *Smell Sweet to God*

The memory verse for this week reminds us that Jesus gave His life as a fragrant offering. The sweet smell Paul alluded to related to the sacrifice of offerings in Old Testament times. The book of Leviticus describes the sacrificial system God instituted in Israel.

➤ Read Leviticus 1:3,10,14. Complete the following statements regarding the three types of offerings to be presented in the Tabernacle:

1. A burnt offering from the _____ was to be a
_____ .

2. A burnt offering from the _____ was to be a
_____ .

3. A burnt offering of a _____ could also be made.

➤ What was the result of each of these three offerings, according to verses 9, 13 and 17?

When the wise men offered the Christ Child the gift of incense (see Matthew 2:11), their gift symbolized the purpose for Christ's coming—His sacrificial death on the cross.

➤ What did Christ have in common with the offerings of the Old Testament?

➤ According to 2 Corinthians 2:14-16, to those who are being saved, Christians are _____ .

➤ To those who are perishing, Christians are _____
_____ .

❧ Do you know any unsaved person who may be depending on you to be a life-giving fragrance? Write that person's name, and then purpose to pray regularly for him or her.

Even our speech might have a way of spreading God's fragrance around us.

❧ According to Ephesians 4:29, what should characterize our speech?

❧ What are some ways your speech can glorify God this week?

❧ Write Proverbs 15:4 in your own words.

Are you sweet smelling to God? Focus this week on making your speech a sweet-smelling aroma to Him. Choose to develop an attitude of thanksgiving and wholesome speech as a way of life.

Holy God, thank You for the sacrifice of Your precious Son, Jesus Christ, as the sweet-smelling offering for the atonement of my sins.

Lord Jesus, help me to use my speech and actions today to be the fragrance of love and hope to those who are perishing without You.

DAY 5: Offer a Sacrifice of Praise

If you haven't memorized Ephesians 5:2 yet, repeat the verse several times now. The last portion of the verse emphasizes Christ's sacrifice for you. You may have also memorized Romans 3:25 as part of the Roman road to salvation.

➤ What is the purpose of the sacrifice as recounted in Romans 3:25?

Yes, Christ was a sacrifice of atonement. Through faith in the blood of Christ for washing away your sin, you accept God's offer of salvation. You cannot offer yourself as a perfect sacrifice for sin. You accept Jesus' sinless life as the only sin offering that counts with God. However, you can demonstrate this same spirit of sacrifice in the way you live.

➤ After reading Hebrews 13:15-16, list the three types of sacrifices you are called upon to offer.

➤ Write your own sacrifice of praise, extolling God's character and virtues.

➤ In Psalm 117, how does David state his praise?

You may think of healthy eating and exercising as sacrifices you make to lose weight, improve your health or become physically fit. You may sacrifice money, time and talent to serve God. Whatever the sacrifice, you will find it to be a fragrant offering to God when you sacrifice out of love.

≫ Describe how you are living a more sacrificial lifestyle in order to achieve your First Place goals.

Heavenly Father, help me today to live a sacrificial life that will be pleasing to You.

Lord Jesus, You offered the ultimate sacrifice for my sins, and I praise and exalt Your name on high in thanksgiving for Your love.

DAY 6: *Reflections*

This week's memory verse admonishes us to live a life of love. That sounds easy until you read the rest of it and realize the love Paul described is a sacrificial love, just like Christ's love for us. Christ expressed His love for each of us with the ultimate sacrifice of His life.

No one in your First Place group will probably ever be called upon to make such a sacrifice, but would you be willing to lay down your life to demonstrate your undying love for Christ? No one knows the exact answer until the moment comes to make such a decision.

Christ doesn't routinely ask for your death to demonstrate love, but He does routinely ask you to sacrifice yourself so that others may see Christ in you. Jesus called His disciples to be a light in a world of darkness and sin. He calls you to the same mission. All He asks is that you obey His commandments and let Him guide your footsteps. You learned how important obedience is to God in Day 1 of your study. How obedient are you to God's command to love others as He has loved you?

In your prayer time, think of the people you listed as needing your forgiveness or of whom you need to ask forgiveness. Search your heart and ask yourself if you have really forgiven in the depths of your heart. No bitterness is to remain. No resentment is to be tucked away in a corner of the heart. It all must be expunged and the person fully forgiven, even as Christ forgives you.

Love is so important to God that it is one of the most often used words in the Bible. Look in the concordance, and you will find pages of Scripture on love. Look up some of the verses and memorize them. Let them be a constant reminder of what God expects of you as you live out the legacy of His love.

Heavenly Father, help to love my enemies and to pray for those who have hurt me and caused me pain (see Matthew 5:44).

Lord Jesus, help me to love as You have loved me and to remain in that love through obedience to Your commands just as You obeyed Your Father and remain in His love (see John 15:9-10).

Father God, I am convinced that neither death nor life, neither angels nor demons, neither the present nor the future, nor any powers, neither height nor depth, not anything else in all creation, will be able to separate me from Your love that is in Christ Jesus, my Lord (see Romans 8:38-39).

DAY 7: *Reflections*

Throughout this study we have been looking at the purposes or reasons for memorizing Scripture. Scripture memory can help us in times of difficulty and give us guidance. Another purpose is to help you draw closer to Him and have a more intimate relationship with Him.

Your closest friends are those with whom you spend time and share your concerns. God wants to be your closest friend. He wants to know all your cares and sorrows, and He wants you to give them all to Him. Many times Christians build barriers between themselves and God and miss out on the close relationship with the best friend they will ever have. What builds those barriers or walls? What in your life might be a stronghold preventing you from enjoying an intimate relationship with your best friend?

In *Praying God's Word*, Beth Moore discusses the many attitudes and feelings a Christian may develop as a stronghold or barrier against intimacy with God. Among them are pride, feeling unloved, feeling rejected, guilt, depression, addiction, unbelief, despair and even food-related barriers. At times, most Christians will experience one or more of the feelings and attitudes that build barriers. Memorizing and praying God's Word will break down those strongholds and bring you into a closer, more intimate relationship with your Lord God.[1]

No matter what the stronghold is, God is bigger and more powerful. Satan will try to make you believe this isn't true, but Satan is a liar and thief. He lies to you to make you doubt, and then he steals your relationship with God. Don't let him get a toehold. Hide God's Word in your heart to use as a weapon that will draw you close to God and far away from Satan.

The following prayer Scriptures will lead you away from Satan and into the presence of God:

I will sing to You, Lord, for You are highly exalted. The horse and its rider You have hurled into the sea! You, Lord, are my strength and my song; You have become my salvation. You are my God and I will praise You. You, Lord, are a warrior! The Lord is Your name! (see Exodus 15:1-3).[2]

Who among the gods is like You, O Lord? Who is like You—majestic in holiness, awesome in glory, working wonders? Stretch out Your right hand and deal with my enemy, O, God! (see Exodus 15:11-12).[3]

I trust in You, O Lord; I say, "You are my God." My times are in Your hands; deliver me from my enemies and those who pursue me. Let Your face shine on Your servant; save me in Your unfailing love. Let me not be put to shame, O Lord, for I have cried out to You (see Psalm 31:14-17).[4]

Mighty God, Your Word clearly states that Satan himself masquerades as an angel of light. Help me to be very discerning because his servants also masquerade as servants of righteousness (see 2 Corinthians 11:14).[5]

Holy Father, help me to live a life of love, just as Christ loved me and gave Himself as a fragrant offering and sacrifice for my sins (see Ephesians 5:2).

Notes
1. Beth Moore, *Praying God's Word* (Nashville, TN: Broadman and Holman, 2000).
2. Ibid., p. 312.
3. Ibid.
4. Ibid., p. 319.
5. Ibid., p. 327.

GROUP PRAYER REQUESTS TODAY'S DATE:_____

NAME	REQUEST	RESULTS

LIVING
IN THE LIGHT

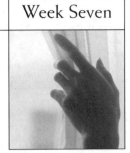

MEMORY VERSE

*You were once darkness,
but now you are light in the Lord.
Live as children of light.*

Ephesians 5:8

Ephesians 5:3-21 contains a series of contrasts. At first glance it seems that Paul concentrated more on the prohibitions for Christians, but when you look beyond the negatives, you see what Christ has freed you from so that you might be His light to this dark world. In this week's study you will examine your heritage as one who shares in His light.

DAY 1: *The Fruit of the Light*

Jesus told a story of the worthlessness of self-reformation. Matthew 12:43-45 is a powerful story of a man who gained temporary freedom from a demon. The man cleaned and swept his house, but he neglected to replace the void left by the fleeing demon with positive things. The demon returned to find his former dwelling cleaned and swept, so he enlisted seven other spirits worse than himself, and they all took up residence! The man's final state was worse than his first.

Like the man in the story, many try to clean their own lives, thinking that somehow they will make themselves acceptable to God. In your attempt to be rid of the negative, do you overlook filling your life with positives? Do you see the darkness, but forget that you are a child of the light?

➤ In Ephesians 5:8-9, what did Paul identify as the fruit of the light?

You cannot generate these characteristics on your own, because this is the fruit that the Holy Spirit has purposed to grow in your life. They are gifts of grace developed through faith and faithfulness.

➤ Which of the three characteristics do you most readily see in yourself?

➤ Which one do you have difficulty identifying in your life?

➤ Identify one step you can take to cultivate these fruits in your life.

➤ What does 2 Corinthians 5:21 say about righteousness?

You are a child of His light, and you have righteousness, goodness and truth through Christ.

 Heavenly Father, I seek Your help and guidance in working out the characteristics of goodness, righteousness and truth in my life.

Thank You, Father God, for sending Jesus Christ to pay for my sin so that I might become the righteousness of God.

DAY 2: *The Fruitless Deeds of Darkness*

You can better appreciate goodness, righteousness and truth when you see them in contrast to the fruitless deeds of darkness.

> ➤ Identify the six fruitless deeds of darkness that appear in Ephesians 5:3-7,11.

In yesterday's study you read the story of the man who cleaned his house but did not replace evil with good. Both Jesus and Paul have told you that the only way to displace evil is to replace it with good.

> ➤ The deeds listed in Ephesians 5:3-5 have infected all the children of Adam. Why are these deeds to be avoided?

These negative characteristics can be displaced with holiness.

> ➤ What does 1 Peter 1:15-16 say about being holy?

Holiness can only be in evidence in a person's life through the presence of God. Holiness is God centered, not human centered.

> ➤ According to Ephesians 5:4, what are the things to be avoided in your speech?

> ➤ With what are they to be replaced?

➤ Paraphrase James 3:9-12.

Lord Jesus, help me to focus on Your holiness rather than on my sins and failures. Help me to seek Your holy presence on a daily basis so that I might begin to be Your light in this dark world.

Heavenly Father, I praise Your name with thanksgiving on my heart for Your bountiful love and mercy. Thank You for Your light in my life.

DAY 3: *The Value of Your Time*

➤ According to Ephesians 5:15-17, what are the three ways to make the most of your time?

The essence of wisdom is to spend time on things of value. The essence of foolishness is to waste time on things that have no value. You will only know what things have value as you understand God's will—what He desires for your life.

➤ Describe the teaching in the parable in Matthew 25:1-13.

➤ What are the similarities between this parable and the message in Ephesians 5:15-17?

When you squander your time on things that do not matter, you are often unprepared for things that do matter, or you may miss valuable time that could be spent on something important.

➤ During the past week, what trivial matters robbed valuable time from the important things on your schedule?

➤ List three occasions when you used your time wisely. (Don't overlook such activities as listening to a child or caring for a friend.)

➤ How do your First Place commitments fit in with using your time wisely?

God gives you the gift of time. You will choose what you do with it. If your schedule seems to overwhelm you at times, submit your schedule to God and let Him direct your decisions about how you will spend your time.

Heavenly Father, help me to be prepared in every area of my life for Your return.

Lord, I submit my time to You. Direct my decisions today as I go about my activities.

DAY 4: *The Filling of the Spirit*

Christians are filled with the Holy Spirit, and when they allow the Spirit to guide their lives, they develop a close relationship with the Father.

⇒ Read Ephesians 5:18; then fill in the following blanks:

Do not get _____ on wine, which leads to
_____. Instead, be _____
with the Spirit.

Alcohol anesthetizes the brain, which makes some people feel free and in control—even though they are losing control. Alcohol gives the illusion of solving problems and escaping reality while actually the problems only grow and become more unmanageable.

The word "debauchery" describes an eroded life. Such a person has been overcome so often that he or she slides easily under the influence of the evil forces. A pattern of drunkenness leads to a broken, wasted, defeated life.

Paul contrasted drunkenness with being filled with the Spirit. What alcohol falsely promises, the Spirit delivers. The Spirit compensates for your weaknesses with God's power. The Spirit empowers you to solve problems so that life becomes manageable.

⇒ Describe a person who is consistently being filled with the Spirit, as noted in Galatians 5:16,22-25.

⇒ According to Galatians 6:8, what is the difference between pleasing the sinful nature and pleasing the Spirit?

The command is "be filled with the Spirit" (Ephesians 5:18). As you keep on being filled, you will develop a life pattern of being strengthened in the Lord and living in His control.

 Heavenly Father, I seek Your strength to help me live my life under Your control.

Lord Jesus, fill me with the Holy Spirit and continue to fill me day by day as I develop a life pattern of strength through You.

DAY 5: A Thankful Heart

➤ What is the outgrowth of being filled with the Spirit, as described in Ephesians 5:19-20?

➤ To whom are you to always give thanks?

Possibly no character trait does more to brighten your life than does a habit of gratitude. Earlier in this study, you were asked to list some of God's blessings in your life. Do you remember to thank God for those blessings in your prayer time? Every day God gives you blessings and reasons to give thanks, even in the face of trial and tragedy.

Three reasons you are grateful today	Three things that challenge your gratefulness today

Look at the two lists. You get to choose which list you will allow to influence your life today. Every day you make decisions—deliberately or by default—that determine the future course of your life. Project yourself into the future and look at your first list.

✎ If you daily choose to be grateful by meditating on the good things, what will be the likely outcome in your character?

✎ If you daily choose to be ungrateful by focusing on the second list, what attitudes will characterize you?

✎ In Philippians 4:4-7, what are the instructions regarding the secret of being at peace with God?

"Rejoice in the Lord always" (v.4). Let Him have your worries and spend a few minutes each day just practicing gratefulness and thanking Him for the little things you normally take for granted. Thank Him for the people who have added to your life and helped you to be a better person or a better friend. Thank Him for Jesus Christ and the Holy Spirit in your life.

Thank You, Heavenly Father, for sending Jesus and giving me an inheritance through Him.

Thank You, Holy Lord, for the little things in life that bring pleasure and happiness every day.

DAY 6: *Reflections*

This week's memory verse is short and easy to memorize, but it also has a profound message for you. Are you living as a child of the light or a child of the darkness? A child of the light will live a life that is markedly different from the life of those who live in the dark. You have gained your freedom from the prince of darkness and have the power of the Holy Spirit and the Light of the world at your disposal.

Goodness, righteousness and truth are the fruits of the life of light and they are given to you by God the Father when you become His child. When goodness, righteousness and truth are the standards by which you live, your relationship with God will grow closer.

Think about the thoughts that fill your mind each day. Are they pleasing to God? Replace the wrong thoughts with words of thanksgiving and praise. Focus on the things that bring truth and light. Make the most of the time God gives you each day, and seek His guidance in all you do.

 Father, I pray that the words of my mouth and the meditations of my heart will be pleasing in Your sight, my Rock and my Redeemer (see Psalm 19:14).

Heavenly Father, I pray my light will shine before men so that they may see good deeds and praise You, my Father in heaven (see Matthew 5:16).

DAY 7: *Reflections*

As a part of living in the light of Jesus Christ, your heart will want to continually praise Him and give thanks for all the many blessings He has given you. That leads to another reason for memorizing Scripture: When God's Word is written in your heart, you will always have words of praise and thanksgiving ready to give Him glory and honor.

The Bible is filled with verses written by men of God who loved Him and praised His name in all situations. David wrote many psalms of adoration and exaltation for the God He knew and loved. Even when David confessed his sins, he never ceased to praise God for His mercy and love.

You, too, can praise God in any and every situation. When you know His Word is true, you can confidently claim His promises. They are a part of the rich inheritance He gives to everyone who calls on His name in repentance of sin.

Use the following Scripture prayers to give thanks and praise to the one true God:

Heavenly Father, I enter Your gates with thanksgiving and come into Your courts with praise; I give thanks to You and praise Your name (see Psalm 100:4).

I will give thanks to You and call on Your name; I will make You known among the nations for what You have done. I will sing praise to You and tell of Your wonderful acts (see Psalm 105:1-2).

My soul will praise Your name, O God; with all my inmost being I will praise Your holy name (see Psalm 103:1).

I was once in darkness, but now I am a light in the Lord. Let me live as a child of the light (see Ephesians 5:8).

GROUP PRAYER REQUESTS   TODAY'S DATE:_____

NAME	REQUEST	RESULTS

THE FAMILY
OF FAITH

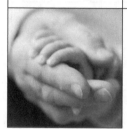

MEMORY VERSE
Make every effort to keep the unity of the Spirit
through the bond of peace.
Ephesians 4:3

Your inheritance in Christ should make an enormous difference in your
relationships. In this week's study you will explore how the message of
Ephesians impacts relationships between believers, wives and husbands,
children and parents, and coworkers.

DAY 1: *Unity Among Believers*

"I don't go to church," the smug young man told the visitor at his apartment
door. "I grew up in a church, and all they did was fight."

Why are Christians often perceived as quarrelsome, arguing over anything from the color of the sanctuary carpet to basic doctrines? Churches
sometimes split over matters that seem to be insignificant years later.
Congregations are torn apart because neither group is willing to compro-
mise and meet the other halfway. This is in direct contradiction to what
God wants for the Church.

➣ What is the key word in Ephesians 4:3 and 4:13?

This word "unity" means "a state of oneness." God puts a high premium
on unity in His family.

❧ What does each of the following Scripture passages say about unity in God's family?

🍎 Psalm 133:1

🍎 John 17:23

🍎 Romans 15:5

❧ What is the ultimate goal of your Christian journey, as stated in Ephesians 4:13?

❧ What is the new command given by Jesus in John 13:34-35?

Notice that Jesus didn't say "all men will know you are my disciples by your perfect, sin-free lifestyle or your perfect families or your incredible self-discipline." The most dramatic demonstration of the Christian life is the unconditional love we show to others.

You undoubtedly know some fellow believers who challenge your ability to love. For some reason they get on your nerves or rub you the wrong way, but they are still God's children. Take time to pray for those who stretch your unity muscles. God will help you grow and mature in His love.

 Heavenly Father, thank You for loving me and giving me the opportunity to grow in Your love and to live by Your commandments.

Holy Lord, I pray for wisdom and a willing spirit to show love to difficult members of my family both at home and in my church.

DAY 2: *Dealing with Anger*

Some people grow up holding in their anger while others seem to let their anger fly no matter who may be around. Frank grew up with the message that anger is wrong or sinful. He prides himself on controlling his anger. Actually, he just stuffs it deep inside. Is it any wonder Frank does not feel very close to anyone?

Sally grew up getting her way by having temper tantrums. Today she lets her anger fly on anyone who happens to be near her. Is it any wonder that no one wants to be around her for very long?

➵ What is the truth found in Ephesians 4:25-32?

It is impossible to never be angry. We will be angry at times—sometimes rightfully so. Even Jesus became angry. He was angered by the money changers and merchants in the Temple and threw them out. He said some harsh things to the Pharisees because of their self-righteousness. We are to speak truthfully, but how we express anger is the issue.

➵ Read the distinctive teachings about anger in each verse of Ephesians 4:25-32; then complete the following statements:

🍎 Verse 26: In your anger, do not_____.

🍎 Verse 31: Get_____of your anger and the_____that it will grow into if you do not deal with it.

🍎 Verse 32: Build on a foundation of_____and _____.

➤ How do you deal with anger? Check all that apply.

☐ I stuff my anger and pretend that I'm not angry.

☐ I stay angry for a long time.

☐ I blow up and then get over my anger; however, my words often hurt others.

☐ I try to honestly express my anger in nondestructive ways.

Let God show you the truth about your anger. He will teach you to deal with your anger in healthy ways. He will give you the courage to feel anger and express it honestly, and in the process He will give you a kind and tender heart.

Heavenly Father, help me to control my anger so that I may be kind and tenderhearted toward my friends.

Lord God, teach me to deal honestly with my anger in healthy ways.

DAY 3: *Wives and Husbands*

In yesterday's study we tackled the difficult subject of anger. Today's lesson moves to the place where anger hits home—how people treat each other in marriage. Remember Paul's instructions: Be honest; be loving; deal with anger and get rid of it.

Perhaps you are not married. The Ephesians passage for today is an analogy for all Christians. It presents marriage as an earthly picture of your heavenly relationship, with you as the bride of Christ and Him the loving Bridegroom. As a Christian you are a member of the family, and the Christian family is the Bride of Christ—His Church.

➤ According to Ephesians 5:21-23, all believers are to ⌣_____
_____to each other out of reverence to Christ.

➤ Wives are to respond to their husbands the way the Church is to

relate to _____.

⋙ Husbands are to respond to their wives the way Christ relates to the

_____.

This passage teaches that marriage partners must treat one another with love and sacrificial service. They are to care for and nurture each other the way they would care for their own bodies. This passage also affirms that our highest allegiance is to Christ. In order for a marriage to function as God designed it, He must be in charge of the home.

⋙ Is Christ the head of your home?

☐ Yes ☐ No

Notice the order in Ephesians. First Paul taught about anger in chapter 4. Then he connected anger and truth—we are to be honest about our anger. Then we are to forgive one another (see Ephesians 4:32) and practice love and submission (see Ephesians 5:21).

⋙ After reading Ephesians 5:29 again, check the statement that most nearly describes how you feel about your body.

☐ I totally accept my body as a gift from God.
☐ I dislike certain aspects of my body, but I accept it as God's gift.
☐ I hate my body.
☐ Other _____

⋙ What could you do to better accept, nourish and care for your body?

God gave you your body to be His temple. Are you doing your best to take care of it as His temple? Be thankful for the body God gives you; then do everything you can to bring honor to Him through your body.

 Heavenly Father, I thank You for the body You gave to me. Help me to take care of it and to use it for Your glory.

Father God, I pray for the wisdom to know how to better relate to others in submission and love, just as You relate to me in love.

DAY 4: *Children and Parents*

Paul admonished us to seek unity in Christ. We find true unity when we practice honesty, love and submission. Now let's apply the quest for unity to parenting issues.

➤ According to Ephesians 6:1-4, what are children to learn?

➤ What is the promised outcome of children learning to obey parents?

➤ What potential problems will children develop if they don't learn to obey their parents?

The reward for children obeying parents is both a promise and a practical result. If children develop a disobedient character, they will have trouble in life. If children learn obedience and self-discipline, "it may go well with" them (v.3). As parents, we are to instill obedience and the resulting self-discipline in our children. The test of discipline is how a child behaves when the parent is out of the room.

➤ What parenting principle is found in verse 4?

The Ten Commandments gave specific instructions about our relationship with our parents, as alluded to in Ephesians 6:2.

⟩⟩ What does Exodus 20:12 say about how we are to treat our parents, and what are we promised when we obey God's instruction?

When parents discipline with love and tenderness rather than with harsh punishment, children will honor their parents. Harsh discipline "exasperates" children, which means "to irritate to the point of anger."

⟩⟩ At this stage in your life, how can you honor *your* parents even if one or both are no longer living?

The behavior of parents in their later years may be erratic, unpredictable and at times exasperating. Remember that you are still their child and honoring them is right in the eyes of the Lord.

 Heavenly Father, I pray for all parents—that they may teach and train their children in Your ways.

Lord, help me to teach my children healthy and honest ways to deal with anger by modeling good behavior and controlling my anger toward them.

DAY 5: *Coworkers*

In Paul's day many people were slaves, so he wrote instructions to slaves and masters. Thankfully, today most people work as employees rather than slaves, but we can still glean practical guidance about the workplace from Paul's letters.

⟩⟩ After reading Ephesians 4:28 and 6:5-9, write the keywords or phrases that apply to the work situation.

➤ Write Ephesians 6:7 in your own words.

➤ Think of how your workplace, your home, your family and your community will be impacted if you choose to see yourself as working for the Lord. If you are a manager, director or supervisor with people under you, what difference should working for Christ have on your attitude toward and treatment of employees?

➤ List the qualities and characteristics from Ephesians 4:2 that you should develop as one called of God.

➤ As you read Ephesians 4:4-6, list the seven unities that Christians must keep.

➤ What impact do these verses have on your daily life?

This week's study has concerned unity. Christ desires unity in His Church. We experience unity when we practice honesty, manage anger, love submissively, serve wholeheartedly and leave the rewards up to the Master.

Heavenly Father, may Your power be in me today as I whole-heartedly serve You.

Lord Jesus, help me to develop the characteristics of gentleness, patience, humility and love as I work with and come into contact with people today. Help me deal with anger in constructive, honest ways.

DAY 6: *Reflections*

In this week's study we have learned about the various aspects of unity. Because of our inheritance in Christ, relationships with the people in our lives will change. A church, family or group of friends cannot exist in harmony unless they have a unity of spirit. When people disagree to the point of alienation, churches split, families are torn apart and friendships dissolve. It is up to you, as a child of God, to do everything you can to bring harmony to your church, your family, your workplace and your friendships.

When the Word of God dwells in you, you can pray and act in a manner that will let others see that you know and love God. Your words will encourage, bring peace and soothe hurt feelings. When the words you speak are words from God in the form of the memory verses you have learned through First Place or on your own, they have much more impact. God's Word gives you His words to use in any circumstance in which you find yourself.

Think about the memory verse for this week. After you memorize it, think of ways you can use it with your family and friends. Think about the peace that comes from being in harmony with God's plan. Pray for your church, your family and your friends to be unified through Christ.

Father, I pray I will keep unity by seeing that no one misses Your grace and that no bitter root grows up to cause problems and defile many (see Hebrews 12:15).

O Lord, may You who gives endurance and encouragement give a spirit of unity among us as we follow the Lord Jesus Christ (see Romans 15:5).

Dear God, over everything that is good, let me put on love which binds us all together in perfect unity (see Colossians 3:14).

DAY 7: *Reflections*

Another purpose for memorizing God's Word is that it will give you comfort and also provide words of encouragement and counsel for others who are in need of prayer and support.

Imagine a friend calling you with a problem or concern on his or her heart. That friend asks you what should be done in a situation or asks you to pray for him or her. Now imagine that you are not able to help because you have nothing to say that will be of any encouragement or comfort. What a terrible feeling! That will not happen when you have the Word of God memorized and ready to use for comfort and encouragement.

In your journal—or wherever you are writing your list of verses to memorize—make a section for Scriptures that give comfort, wisdom, encouragement and counsel. Look up the words in a concordance and find Scripture references for these terms. Then find the Scriptures and read them to see if they fit the category and will be of help to you and to others who need comfort or encouragement.

Make the verses yours by using first person pronouns and by using your own name in appropriate places. Write the verses; then repeat the verses several times. Write them again without looking at the references. Do this several times, and then find someone to whom you can say the verses. Soon you will discover the verses are written on your heart. What a privilege it is to then be able to call the verses to mind when a friend is in need.

The following verses can be used for your own comfort and encouragement or for others:

 O Lord, You will guide me always; You will satisfy my need in a sun-scorched land, and You will strengthen my body so that I will be like a well-watered garden, like a spring whose waters never fail (see Isaiah 58:11).

Heavenly Father, I will lie down and sleep in peace, for You alone, O Lord, make me dwell in safety (see Psalm 4:8).

In You, O Lord, my soul finds rest. My hope is in You alone. You alone are my rock and my salvation; You are my fortress, I will not be shaken (see Psalm 62:5).

Father God, I will make every effort to keep the unity of the Spirit through the bond of peace (see Ephesians 4:3).

GROUP PRAYER REQUESTS   TODAY'S DATE:_____

NAME	REQUEST	RESULTS

THE WINNING SIDE

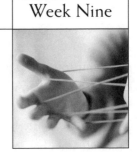

MEMORY VERSE

Our struggle is not against flesh and blood,
but against the rulers, against the authorities,
against the powers of this dark world and against
the spiritual forces of evil in the heavenly realms.
Ephesians 6:12

Many people live in war-torn countries. There are many accounts of the horrors of prisoner-of-war camps where prisoners are often tortured physically, mentally and emotionally in ways beyond description. Those who survive live with external and internal scars.

The apostle Paul knew firsthand the experience of being a prisoner. He had been beaten, and his ankles and wrists were chained. Still, he could say the struggles against flesh and blood are nothing compared to spiritual warfare. In the fight against darkness, God's army takes on Satan's formidable forces, and yes, Satan takes prisoners here on Earth! Fortunately, we know that ultimately we are on the winning side.

We have spent several weeks focusing on the transforming benefits of our precious inheritance from God the Father. But now the mood of discussion changes. In this week's study we will discover ways Satan tries to keep us from claiming our legacy in Christ.

DAY 1: *Your Worst Enemy*

You can be a believer, a soldier of the Lord's army, and still be imprisoned by Satan in slavery to sin. American prisoners of the Vietcong were no less American because they were POWs. The enemy could not take their citizenship away, but the Vietcong attempted to strip them of their dignity and all that made them effective soldiers and human beings.

Considering Ephesians 6:12, list the adversaries with whom we struggle.

Our toughest struggles are not with family members, friends, work associates or even with eating habits or inactive lifestyles. Our toughest battle is against the power of darkness and Satan, the prince of darkness. Sometimes he disguises himself in the difficulties that you may have with a family member or a lifestyle issue. But make no mistake about it, Satan is at the heart of any struggle you experience.

Describe an area in your life in which you are convinced that Satan was at the root of a battle.

How did you attempt to defeat the enemy in this situation?

Satan would like nothing better than to blot from your memory the fact that you are a totally accepted, completely forgiven child of God. Do not let him rob you of the victorious life you have in Christ. God will rescue you out of every situation when you daily call on Him for help and guidance. He will give you the victory.

In Galatians 1:3-5, Paul wrote a greeting to the church and its members. What is the promise in this passage?

Thank You, Lord God, for giving me a victorious life over sin through Your Son, Jesus Christ.

Heavenly Father, I ask for Your strength to give me the power to resist my enemy, Satan, every day of my life.

DAY 2: *What Satan Wants*

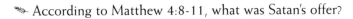

When Satan tempts or thwarts you, what is his ultimate intention? Is it just to make your day a little more miserable, or does he have a more sinister purpose?

➤ According to Matthew 4:8-11, what was Satan's offer?

➤ What were Satan's conditions?

➤ What was Christ's response?

➤ In your own words, explain Satan's purpose in tempting you.

The worship of Satan is alive and well in American society! He wants everyone to worship him instead of God. When you give Satan a place of influence in your life, he has scored a victory against his chief rival, our Creator and Sovereign Lord. However, we need to remember who has the ultimate power to be victorious.

≫ According to Ephesians 6:10-11, on whose strength and power are we to rely?

Before attempting to combat the enemy on your own, realize that nowhere in Scripture are you promised victory over temptation through your own willpower or self-discipline. Only through the intervention of our Commander in Chief, the Lord God, will the victory be won.

≫ What does Colossians 1:16 assure you about God?

≫ Is there anything over which God is not superior?

☐ Yes   ☐ No

God is the creator of everything in heaven and on Earth. That gives Him superiority over all things. No one—not even invisible demonic powers—can claim authority over Him. He has power and strength in your life. He is your Lord and worthy of all worship and praise. Stand in His presence and be amazed at all He can do for you.

Thank You, Heavenly Father, for the power and strength You give me to resist temptations placed before me by my enemy, Satan.

Lord God, You alone are my God, and I worship You and praise Your name. Let Your name be exalted above all the earth.

DAY 3: *What Defeats the Devil*

Although you cannot defeat Satan through your own power, God does expect your cooperation in the battle! You cannot sit on the sidelines and pretend to be neutral. God's strength and power, together with your active participation in God's plan, will overcome temptation.

➤ Read 1 Peter 5:8-9. Describe your role in Satan's defeat by filling in the following blanks:

🍎 Be _____ and _____.

🍎 Resist him, _____
   in the faith.

➤ Why do you need to be careful?

A sentinel must be alert at all times, on the lookout for enemy troops. Alertness characterizes a Christian who does not want temptation to sneak up on him or her.

Note that you effectively resist Satan when you stand firm in your faith. Times of doubt or discouragement make you vulnerable to temptation. God is with you every time you do battle with Satan or encounter him.

➤ What advice in 1 Peter 5:7 should be remembered and followed daily?

Turn all your cares, worries and temptations over to God every day.

Lord God, I give You my life today and trust You to take care of all my worries, fears and temptations.

Heavenly Father, help me today to be self-controlled and alert to the temptations Satan puts in my path.

DAY 4: *Playing into His Hands*

Persons who want to be victorious over Satan must refuse to give him an advantage. Paul warned the Christians in Corinth that they were in danger of doing just that. The believers at Corinth were refusing to forgive and comfort a sinner who needed their love and compassion.

➤ What did Paul say about forgiveness in 2 Corinthians 2:10-11?

➤ Why would unforgiveness enable Satan to outwit believers?

Unforgiveness gives Satan direct advantage! It ties us to the past and problems, and it brings us pain. Many times in our lives we will have people who hurt or disappoint us so terribly that it is hard to forgive them.

➤ Who or what needs to be forgiven in your life?

One of Satan's favorite schemes is to keep you bound to your past. As long as you focus on your hurt, Satan will keep you in his grip. Remember the story of Martha and her brother from week five? As long as she didn't forgive her brother, she let all the past pain fill her life and keep her from a closer relationship not only with her brother but also with God. Satan loves situations like this. He wants the pain and hurt to eat at you and spoil your relationships so that you are unable to fully realize God's power and plan for you in the present and in the future.

➤ Have you experienced the truth of John 8:36?

☐ Yes   ☐ No

God seeks to set you free through the blood of Jesus Christ.

➤ According to Galatians 5:1, why were you set free?

Slavery to the past, like slavery to sin, imprisons you. Christ died that you may never again be imprisoned by Satan!

➤ What in your lifestyle binds you and holds you back? Check all that apply.

☐ Poor eating habits

☐ Lack of exercise

☐ Substances (caffeine, nicotine, alcohol) that harm my body

☐ Lack of sleep

☐ Poor stress management

☐ An unresolved problem in a relationship

☐ Inconsistent quiet time for prayer and Bible study

☐ Other _____

 Heavenly Father, help me to rid my life of any of these hindrances so that I may experience the freedom You desire for me.

Lord God, give me a willing spirit to seek Your freedom and victory over Satan.

DAY 5: *And the Winner Is*

If you were commanding an army, would knowing from the beginning that you would win be helpful to you? Talk about confident troops!

Well, we do know the ultimate ending of the battle—the Lord will be the victor.

➤ According to Philippians 2:10-11, why will God triumph over Satan?

≫ Whose name will be exalted?

≫ According to Revelation 20:1-2,7-10, how will Satan be destroyed?

≫ According to 2 Corinthians 10:4, what kinds of weapons are available to you?

≫ Since you know Christ is the ultimate victor, check the feelings that are appropriate for you to have as a believer.

☐ Confidence   ☐ Fear

☐ Assurance   ☐ Boldness

☐ Resistance   ☐ Anxiety

≫ What is the promise found in 1 John 4:4?

With a promise like this, you have nothing to fear. Christ has defeated Satan. Jesus said that He came to give you abundant life in opposition to the one who steals, kills and destroys life. You stand before God as a victorious child of the King. You can boldly go into battle against Satan and confront his temptations.

Thank You, Father God, for giving me a spirit of courage and not of fear.

I stand before You today, Heavenly Father, as a victorious child because You give me the strength and power to defeat Satan.

DAY 6: *Reflections*

Isn't it great to know you are on the winning side? You do not have to fight your battles alone. God is with you and equips you to do battle with Satan every day. This is the battle God wins for you.

Romans 8:38-39 assures us that nothing can separate us from the love of God. No matter what happens, we still have God on our side.

In *Praying God's Word*, Beth Moore devotes an entire chapter to discussing the power God gives us to overcome the enemy and any strongholds. The Word of God and prayer together make a weapon so strong that even Satan flees in fear. As Moore says, "God has handed us two sticks of dynamite with which to demolish our strongholds: His Word and prayer."[1] The following prayers are adapted from her book:

O God, how I thank You for seeing my misery and hearing my cries because of Satan, the slave driver. You are concerned about my suffering. Come down to rescue me, O Lord, and bring me to the place of Your promise (see Exodus 3:7-8).[2]

Lord God, when Your children, the Israelites, were defeated in battle, You revealed to them that they were hanging on to something that did not belong to them. You said, "You cannot stand against your enemies until you remove it" (Joshua 7:13). Father God, I earnestly ask You to reveal anything in my life that could be hindering victory, then give me the courage to release it to You.[3]

Keep me safe, O God, for in You I take refuge. I say to You, Lord, "You are my Lord; apart from you I have no good thing" (Psalm 16:1-2).[4]

Lord, my God, show the wonder of Your great love, You who save by Your right hand those who take refuge in You from their foes. Keep me as the apple of Your eye; hide me in the shadow of Your wings from the wicked who assail me (see Psalm 17:7-9).[5]

Another purpose for memorizing Scripture is to help us teach others about God's love and grace toward them. You may not teach a Sunday School class or lead a Bible study, but you often talk with others—both Christians and non-Christians. God has given you His Word "for teaching, rebuking, correcting and training in righteousness" (2 Timothy 3:16).

Your church has many areas of service in which you can use the Scriptures you memorize to help others know Him. Teaching in Vacation Bible School or Sunday School gives you the opportunity to share God's Word with children. They love learning about Jesus and the Bible. Or perhaps you might volunteer in the library and help people find books and references to help them study the Bible. Knowing God's Word will give you an opportunity to share with others as they seek to know God's truth in their own lives.

The Bible is a rich treasure box full of God's love, mercy and goodness for His children. Use His Word to tell others what He has done for you. Teach them about His ways and guide them into a better understanding of His Word.

We have discussed how people may worship Satan instead of God and how the devil is always on the prowl looking for victims. Many of the people who worship Satan have never heard the real truth about him and about God. They may just need to hear God's truth from someone like you who has God's Word in his or her heart. Even if you feel you are inadequate and lack the skills for teaching, you can still tell others about Him. Open up your mind to God's Word; then open up your heart to those who need to know about Him and His Word. He will be with you and bring to mind the Scriptures you need. The following Scripture prayers will strengthen and guide you in your witness to those who are lost:

Father God, let me study so that I may be a workman who does not need to be ashamed and help me to correctly handle the word of truth (see 2 Timothy 2:15).

O Lord, let me proclaim what I have seen and heard so that others may also have fellowship with You through Jesus Christ (see 1 John 1:3).

Thanks be to You, O God, who always leads me in triumphal procession in Christ and through me spreads everywhere the fragrance of the knowledge of Him (see 2 Corinthians 2:14).

Lord God, I know that if I give, it will be given to me. A good measure, pressed down, shaken together and running over, will be poured into my lap. For with the measure I use, it will be measured to me (see Luke 6:38).

Lord, I know my struggle is not against flesh and blood but against the rulers, against the authorities, against the powers of this dark world and against the spiritual forces of evil in the heavenly realms (see Ephesians 6:12).

Notes

1. Beth Moore, *Praying God's Word* (Nashville, TN: Broadman and Holman, 2000), p. 6.
2. Ibid., p. 312.
3. Ibid., pp. 313-314.
4. Ibid., p. 314.
5. Ibid.

GROUP PRAYER REQUESTS   TODAY'S DATE:_____

NAME	REQUEST	RESULTS

KEEP ON PRAYING

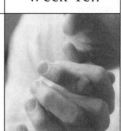

MEMORY VERSE
*Pray in the Spirit on all occasions with
all kinds of prayers and requests.*
Ephesians 6:18

In order to claim the full measure of your inheritance, you need to keep in touch with your Benefactor! God's blessings and protections are best appropriated through prayer. Prayer was God's idea! Jesus gave you a model prayer; Paul was a man of prayer, and he encouraged believers to pray. During this final week of the study, let prayer characterize your relationship with God.

DAY 1: *Pray in the Spirit*

Paul's encouragement to pray in the Spirit followed his detailed description of the armor believers must wear in order to be protected from the devil's schemes. You may have taken a course in self-defense, where you learned certain movements to ward off an attacker. God's Word tells us that self-defense is not enough. We need God's armor and His weapon, the Word of God. Paul concluded this teaching with the admonition to pray.

>>> In Ephesians 6:13-17, what are the last two pieces of your defense (v. 17) against Satan?

>>> Why do you think Paul left these two until the end?

Like any army, faithful followers must get their battle instructions from the commander in chief. Prayer is the channel that keeps you attuned to God's strategy for victory over sin and temptation.

⟿ Consider this week's memory verse—what do you think Paul means by "pray in the Spirit"?

    ☐ Pray as though you were thinking God's very thoughts.

    ☐ Pray when you feel particularly spiritual.

    ☐ Pray, calling on the Spirit to intercede for you.

Paul cancelled out the second option because he said you are to pray "on all occasions." You cannot be guided by feelings or emotions. A pastor told his congregation, "When you don't feel like praying, is when you need it the most."

⟿ In Romans 8:26, what is the role of the Spirit during your prayers?

Heavenly Father, as I pray in the Spirit, reveal to me those weaknesses with which I am going to need help today.

    Holy Lord, thank You for the power of prayer in my life through the Holy Spirit.

DAY 2: *Kinds of Prayers*

How would you feel if your spouse or a child talked to you only if he or she had a need? Eventually, you might think you were only important as a source of money or services. Does God ever feel this way about your relationship with Him?

Prayers should be as varied as your conversations with loved ones. A simple formula for balancing your prayer life is the acrostic *ACTS: A* for adoration or praise, *C* for confession, *T* for thanksgiving and *S* for supplication (requests).

❧ Read the following Bible prayers and then label them with the correct letter from the acrostic ACTS:

_____ Psalm 17:6-8   _____ Psalm 113

_____ Psalm 51:1-4   _____ Psalm 118:1

Although you need to balance your prayer life, you should never hesitate to bring the smallest matter to God in prayer. One elderly Christian woman had such a close relationship with God that she knew He'd answer even the simplest of prayers. One day she became particularly stressed because she had to take her daughter to the airport, and her car keys were nowhere to be found. After 15 minutes of searching, she decided God knew where the keys were. She went into her bedroom, sat on the side of the bed and bowed her head. She simply said, "Lord, You know what I have to do, and You know where the keys are. Please show me." She sat there a few more minutes then said, "Thank You, Jesus." She went back to the kitchen and straight to the cabinet where the keys lay hidden in a coffee cup on a shelf. She believed God, and He answered her.

❧ Paraphrase what Jesus said in Matthew 10:29-31 to prove that God cares about every aspect of your life.

❧ How do you feel about bringing your requests to God? Check all that apply.

☐ I believe He cares about my concerns.
☐ I feel unworthy of His attention.
☐ I try not to bother Him with little things.
☐ I'm thankful that I have God to rely on when I'm trying to make a tough decision.

Claim God's desire and ability to meet your needs. Spend extra time today praising and thanking Him for His provision and protection.

Thank You, Father, for providing for my needs through the riches of Your Son, Jesus Christ.

Thank You, Father God, for being the One to whom I can go when I am in need, whether the problem is large or small. Nothing is insignificant to You.

DAY 3: *The Role of Intercession*

Intercession is one of the great privileges of prayer. If you keep a prayer journal as part of your daily quiet time, you have a record of your prayers. It is a place to record the answers to specific prayers. What could be more satisfying than to write "ANSWERED" across a request?

Prayer journals also show you the focus of your prayers. Is your journal full of me, myself and I? How often do you pray for others? Do you pray for persons you don't know personally? Do you pray for those who live far away, perhaps in another country? Do you pray for others when your prayers will not benefit you in any tangible way?

In this week's memory verse, we are encouraged to keep praying for other Christians with "all kinds of prayers and requests."

➤ Write the names of some Christians outside your family for whom you regularly pray.

Pray for others in order to guard against self-centeredness and spiritual isolation. Pray for others because prayer works! When God wants to do something in the world, He moves people to pray for it. Your greatest privilege is to pray on behalf of others.

➤ Who did the praying in Acts 12:5,12-17?

➤ What did they pray for?

➣ What were the results of their prayers?

God is faithful, even when you lack faith. Ask God to bring to your mind those for whom you need to be praying, including your First Place group.

Thank You, Heavenly Father, for the privilege of prayer and Your promise to answer those who call on Your name and believe in Your Word.

Lord God, I lift up the names of my friends and family and ask Your blessings on them today.

DAY 4: *Prayer for Courage*

When you think of Paul, do you think of a bold witness for Christ? Paul was one of the first Christian missionaries. He described himself as Christ's slave and willingly gave up his freedom and eventually his life in service to his Lord. Would it surprise you to learn that Paul asked for prayers for boldness?

➣ According to Acts 21:10-14, what was Paul's reasoning for going to Jerusalem despite being warned against it?

➣ Read Ephesians 6:19-20. Write Paul's prayer request in your own words.

Like us, Paul had a human nature that responded with fear when he depended on his own resources. He needed the believers' prayers.

≫ What is the source of boldness found in 1 Timothy 1:12?

It takes courage to make changes in your life, to stand up against peer pressure and to defeat temptation.

≫ Describe a time when God gave you courage to make a good decision regarding keeping your First Place commitments.

We do not know specifically why Paul prayed for boldness on this occasion, but we do know he was in chains in prison. Paul knew he needed a fresh blessing of courage to deal with his circumstances. The Holy Spirit will help you know what to pray for if you will ask Him.

≫ What is the promise found in John 16:13?

Let the Holy Spirit guide you today as you pray the following Scripture prayers:

I pray now for the Holy Spirit to guide me in my prayers today and bring to mind those for whom I need to pray.

Thank You, Heavenly Father, for the love You show me through the death of Jesus Christ who paid my debt of sin.

DAY 5: *Undying Love*

Why is it important to communicate regularly with your family members? Counselors tell us that communication is the lifeline of a relationship; couples who do not talk to each other drift apart.

Prayer is your communication lifeline to God. One of the key purposes of prayer is to build a personal love relationship with the Father. Like embers in a fireplace, love must be rekindled in order to keep from dying. You must "pray continually" to nurture your love relationship with God.

➤ In 1 Thessalonians 5:16-18, what three things did Paul tell Christians to do?

➤ Are these things a part of your life? If not, what you can do to bring the joy, prayer and thanksgiving that you need into your life?

➤ What blessing did Paul give those who love God with undying love, as seen in Ephesians 6:23-24?

As this study began, you read about the priceless inheritance of eternal life that now is yours. You learned about the grace that made this unmerited gift possible. When you experience grace, you can extend it to others.

➤ Describe a grace-filled person. If you want this description to characterize your life, sign your name underneath what you write.

➤ If this study has made a difference in your life in terms of how you live your First Place commitments, check the responses that apply.

　☐ I am more aware than ever that my body is the temple of the Holy Spirit, and I am taking better care of it now.

- ☐ I endeavor to seek God's will for my life, including how I spend my time and how I balance work and rest.

- ☐ I recognize how easily I fall victim to Satan's snare. I am becoming more vigilant against temptation, including the temptation to eat unhealthy foods.

- ☐ I now see that I must bathe everything I do in prayer, including lifestyle choices.

- ☐ I claim the peace that is part of my precious inheritance. I pledge to follow Christ's example by making peace wherever I can, including within myself, recognizing that Christ has forgiven me and I can forgive others.

Ideally, you should check all of the statements. Perhaps you can think of others you might want to add in the margins. Tell Jesus how you feel about your legacy and what you hope to accomplish as a result of this study.

Heavenly Father, I give You my undying love and seek Your guidance in all that I do.

Father God, thank You for the legacy You give to all those who believe in Jesus Christ as their personal Savior. Help me to live in such a way that I give Christ first place in every area of my life.

DAY 6: *Reflections*

The focus for this week's session has been prayer. Prayer is your method of communication with God. His line is always open, and He is ready to listen. He cares about you. One of the ways God provides for your needs is through Christian friends who pray for you and minister to you. In return, you pray for them and minister to their needs.

On Day 2 you learned about the acrostic *ACTS* which stands for Adoration, Confession, Thanksgiving and Supplication. When you pray in this way, you include every aspect of prayer as taught and modeled by Jesus. Each is an important step in prayer. However, many times you will simply pray words from the depths of your heart that follow no order or pattern. Even more wonderful is the fact that God knows your needs, and in those times when you are so overcome you can't put your needs into words, God hears, knows and understands.

The most important aspect of prayer is not the order or pattern of your prayer, but that you pray consistently, on all occasions and with all kinds of requests. This is what Paul told the church at Ephesus.

Prayer gets you ready for battle. As stated on Day 1, it is the channel that keeps you attuned to God's strategy for victory over sin and temptation. Remember, when you use the sword of the Spirit—the Word of God—and you pray, your enemy Satan cannot stand up against the power of these two weapons.

 Father God, You have put a new song in my mouth. Praise to God; many will see and fear and will trust in You, O Lord (see Psalm 40:3).

O Lord, You promised to be near me when I have a broken heart and to save me when I have a contrite spirit. Many are my afflictions; but You, Lord, will deliver me out of them all (see Psalm 34:18-19).

You, Eternal God, are my refuge, and underneath me are Your everlasting arms; You will thrust out my enemies from before me and will destroy them (see Deuteronomy 33:27).

You, O Lord, have set me free. I stand firm in that freedom. I will never again be burdened again by the yoke of slavery (see Galatians 5:1).

DAY 7: *Reflections*

You have learned what a rich inheritance you have in Christ—an inheritance that no one can take away from you. God's amazing grace will always be with you, and you are on the winning side in the battle against Satan.

Memorizing Scripture will help you overcome fears, worries and doubts that come into your life. Having the Word of God in your heart brings you the words you need in any situation. God's Word will even teach you how not to worry about the things over which you have no control.

Many overwhelming situations come into your life, but God is faithful; His Word is true. When you know you have no control, give control to God, and He will guide you every step of the way.

When Mary was diagnosed with cancer and faced surgery, she claimed God's promise and turned her cancer over to Him. She amazed friends with her calmness and joy in the face of a life-threatening situation. Her response to their questions was "I've given this to God, and now it's His problem, not mine. I sure can't fix it, but He gave me doctors who know what to do. God will provide for me out of His great riches through Jesus Christ." She held on to that verse from Philippians 4:19. Today she is a cancer survivor.

Since God takes care of the sparrow and the lilies of the field, He will take care of You. Memorize His Word, and you will have a rich treasure of resources to use in your time of need, when worry, fear or other concerns threaten your relationship with God.

The following Scripture prayers address worry, fear and concern:

You, O Lord, are my light and salvation. Whom shall I fear? You are the stronghold of my life; of whom shall I be afraid? (see Psalm 27:1-2).

Heavenly Father, I don't have to be anxious about anything, for I have made my requests known to You by my prayers and supplications. Your peace, which surpasses all understanding will guard my heart and mind through Jesus Christ (see Philippians 4:6-7).

Lord God, I cast all my cares on You, for You will sustain me and will never let me fall (see Psalm 55:22).

Lord Jesus, I will pray in Your Spirit on all occasions with all kinds of prayers and requests (see Ephesians 6:18).

GROUP PRAYER REQUESTS   TODAY'S DATE:_____

NAME	REQUEST	RESULTS

EXERCISING OUTDOORS

One of the best ways to get active is to get out and enjoy God's beautiful creation. There are many enjoyable and beneficial activities you can do outdoors, such as walking, hiking, bicycling, swimming and other recreational sports. However, when it comes to exercising outdoors, there are several things you can do to increase the enjoyment and safety of the activities you choose. It's important to consider weather, clothing, equipment and environment when exercising outdoors. Also, some activities such as downhill skiing, in-line skating and bicycling are more risky and require more precautions for safety. Choose activities you enjoy, but *take it slow and play it smart!*

TIPS FOR EXERCISING SAFELY OUTDOORS

When exercising outdoors, there are several things you need to keep in mind to prevent injury or illness.

What to Wear

A good pair of shoes is the most important piece of equipment for exercising outdoors. Here are some tips for selecting a pair of exercise shoes.

- The best shoe is the one that fits your foot well, not necessarily the most expensive. Try on several pairs before buying. Does the shoe feel natural when you walk? Keep trying until you find one that feels right!

- Make sure the shoe supports your arch and has plenty of room for your toes; allow for a thumb's width between your toes and the end of the shoe. Keep your toenails trimmed!

- For walking or jogging, choose a flexible shoe with good cushioning. Don't go hiking in tennis shoes; wear the appropriate boot or shoe.

- For court and field sports, consider a high-top shoe to protect your ankles.

🍎 Wear cotton or nylon athletic socks. It's not necessary to wear a double layer of socks.

When deciding what clothing to wear, consider the weather and light conditions.

🍎 Whether exercising in the heat or cold, always wear clothing that can be layered and easily removed or put back on as your body temperature changes.

🍎 Check with a local sports store for the best clothing and protective gear for your activity.

🍎 Wear reflective and light-colored clothing, and carry a flashlight at dusk or at night.

🍎 Consider carrying a small backpack or fanny pack to store extra clothing.

🍎 When exercising in the heat, avoid clothing that does not ventilate well, such as rubberized suits or sweatsuits. This is a dangerous practice that can lead to dehydration and heat stroke!

Weather

Extreme temperatures affect how your body responds to exercise. High temperatures and humidity or cold temperatures and wind place additional stress on your body. Check the weather forecast before heading outdoors. *Always decrease your intensity level and take it slow when it's very hot or cold!*

Tips for Beating the Heat

🍎 It's a hot day when the temperature is above 85 degrees or when the temperature plus the humidity is greater than 130 (i.e., 80 degrees + 55% humidity = 135).

🍎 It takes 10 to 14 days to adapt to the heat. If you're exercising in hot conditions, cut your intensity and duration in half and gradually increase your activity as your body adapts to the heat.

🍎 Drink water before, during and after exercise. Drink at least five to eight ounces of cool water 15 minutes before and then every 15 to 20 minutes during exercise.

- On really hot days, exercise during the coolest part of the day or exercise indoors.
- Wear lightweight, loose-fitting clothes, a hat and sunscreen to protect you from the sun. If you wear a hat, make sure it allows for ventilation.

Tips for Exercising Safely in the Cold

- Don't just rely on the thermometer; the wind chill greatly increases the risk of exercising in the cold.
- Dress warmly and in layers that can be easily removed. Several layers warm better than one heavy jacket. Because physical activity quickly generates body heat, it's important to be able to remove layers as your body heats up.
- Wool and synthetic fabrics are good choices because they whisk moisture away from your body. Wear an outer layer that keeps out the wind and moisture.
- Much of your body's heat can be lost through your head and neck, so wear a hat and scarf. Don't forget to protect your hands too.
- Watch out for slick surfaces caused by rain and snow.
- It's just as important to drink water in the cold as in the heat.
- When exercising in the cold, stay close to home or other shelter.

A Note About Altitude

Altitude increases the stress of physical activity. It's harder for your body to take in oxygen above 5,000 feet. This means your heart, lungs and muscles have to work harder. Symptoms of altitude sickness include light-headedness, dizziness, nausea and unusual shortness of breath. Give yourself a couple of days to adjust to the higher elevation, and cut back the intensity of your activities.

THE CHALLENGE TO CHANGE

Change is never easy. In fact, most people successful in changing a lifestyle habit make several attempts before reaching their goal. Few people are successful on their first try. Studies reveal that people who have successfully quit smoking attempted to stop three to four times before achieving their goal. The key is to keep trying; if you really want to change; you can do it. The following statistics reveal how difficult it is to make lasting changes in lifestyle habits:

- 🍎 Over 50 percent of people who start an exercise program drop out within the first three to six months.
- 🍎 Nearly 95 percent of people who lose weight gain it all back within three to five years.
- 🍎 Less than 30 percent of people who make a New Year's resolution stick with it to the end of the year.
- 🍎 Only 30 percent of people who attempt to stop smoking are successful.

The keys to successful lifestyle change are staying on track when times get tough and bouncing back after a setback. The only way to succeed is to realize that you will be tempted and experience setbacks along the way. If you plan ahead and don't have unrealistic expectations, you can reach your goals.

Overcoming Temptation

Have you ever been working toward a goal or maybe even achieved your goal, only to have something come along and knock you off course and put you back right where you started? When making lifestyle changes, such as losing weight or starting an exercise program, people report several situations or factors that often knock them off track. It's important to understand what things will make it difficult for you to achieve your goals. Do any of these sound familiar to you?

≫ In what ways are you likely to be tempted?

- ☐ Stress and other emotional factors
- ☐ Illness or injury (to self or a loved one)
- ☐ Holidays and special occasions
- ☐ The influence of others
- ☐ Overwork
- ☐ Bad weather
- ☐ Travel and vacations

Once you understand how you're likely to be tempted and where your challenges are going to come from, you can begin building a plan that won't allow these situations to knock you off course. Don't let temptation, challenges and setbacks keep you from achieving your goals. When it comes to your health, happiness and quality of life, don't let anything come between you and your goals—that is, if your goals are in line with God's desire for your life. Don't let guilt, negative thinking, embarrassment, feelings of failure, temporary setbacks or any other thing come between you and a worthwhile goal. For encouragement, read Romans 8:28-39. The choice is up to you: You can view setbacks and slipups as failures, or you can view them as learning opportunities to help you grow stronger.

When it comes to making lifestyle changes, you *will* be tempted. Read the account of the temptation of Eve in Genesis 3:1-6. Look at all the dimensions in which she was tempted:

- 🍎 "You will not surely die . . . you will be like God" (spiritual)
- 🍎 "The woman saw that the food was pleasing" (emotional)
- 🍎 "Desirable for gaining wisdom" (intellectual)
- 🍎 "She took some and ate it" (physical)
- 🍎 "She also gave some to her husband" (social)

≫ According to Mark 12:29-30, in what dimensions of your life are you to love God?

Don't get discouraged when you are tempted. God will provide you with a way out (see 1 Corinthians 10:13). If you look for the way out and are willing to act on what God provides, you can overcome temptation. One of the best ways to overcome temptation is to rely on God's Word (see Psalm 119:11; Matthew 4:1-11). Build a list of memory verses that you can hide in your heart to help you through temptation and difficult times.

A Lesson on Learning

The Great Commandment calls you to love God with all your mind. When making lifestyle changes, it's important to learn from both your successes and failures. If you have set a worthwhile goal, it's important to do all you can to achieve success. When you are tempted or you experience a setback, think about what went wrong. Explore ways you can prevent it from happening next time. Ask yourself if your expectations and feelings are realistic. Most importantly, avoid negative thinking. Work through the following exercise to help you learn how to anticipate and deal with temptation and setbacks:

- Think about two similar situations in the past: One in which you were highly tempted but did not give in and one in which you gave in to a temptation that was not consistent with your goals.
- Can you identify a strategy or technique you used in the first situation that you didn't use in the second?
- How did you feel after each situation? Did you feel better about yourself in the first situation? Why?
- What were your feelings when you gave in to temptation?
- Did you feel disappointed, angry or guilty? Why? Were these negative feelings or thoughts realistic? Were they helpful to you? What can you do to keep from feeling disappointed, guilty or having other negative thoughts or feelings the next time you slip up or experience a setback? How can you avoid giving in to temptation next time?

THE
FAITH FACTOR

Recent polls indicate that most Americans believe in the healing power of faith and prayer.

- 🍎 Nearly 80 percent believe that faith, religious practice and personal prayer can speed or help the medical treatment of people who are ill.

- 🍎 More than 77 percent believe that God sometimes intervenes to cure people who have a serious illness.

- 🍎 Over 60 percent say that religion and daily prayer are very important in their life.

- 🍎 Sixty percent say they pray for their own health, and over 80 percent say they pray for the health of others.

Faith and prayer are good for the body, mind and soul. Recent research suggests that faith is an important factor in the prevention of disease and the promotion of health. According to recent scientific evidence, over 78 scientific studies show that religious commitment is beneficial to health and well-being.

A 1997 study of 5,000 men and women found that those who attended religious services frequently were 25 percent less likely to die over 28 years of follow-up as those who attended less frequently. They were also more likely to quit smoking, increase exercise, increase social contacts and have better marriages.

One study found that people who attend church regularly have 50 percent less risk of dying from heart disease and 56 percent less risk of dying from lung disease compared to those who rarely go to church. They also had 74 percent less risk of dying from liver disease and 53 percent less risk of dying from suicide.

Several studies show that faith has beneficial effects on blood pressure. A study of over 4,000 people aged 65 and older found that those who attended religious services at least once a week and prayed or studied the Bible at least daily had consistently lower blood pressure than those who did so less frequently or not at all.

One study found that older patients who attended religious services once a week or more cut their risk of being hospitalized in the previous year by 56 percent compared to patients who attended less frequently. Hospitalized patients with a religious affiliation cut their hospital stay in half compared to those without an affiliation.

The following questions are similar to the types of questions asked in the research studies previously discussed. Research suggests that the lower your score on each of these questions, the more positive is the impact of your Christian faith on your health and well-being.

➤ How often do you attend church or other worship services?

☐ More than once a week   ☐ Once a week

☐ A few times a month   ☐ A few times a year

☐ Once a year or less   ☐ Never

➤ How often do you spend time in personal religious activities, such as prayer, meditation and Bible study?

☐ More than once a day   ☐ Daily

☐ Two or more times a week   ☐ Once a week

☐ A few times a month   ☐ Rarely or never

➤ My Christian faith is what lies behind my whole approach to life.

☐ Definitely true of me   ☐ Tends to be true

☐ Unsure   ☐ Tends not to be true

☐ Definitely not true

➤ I try hard to carry my Christian faith over into all other dealings in my life.

☐ Definitely true of me   ☐ Tends to be true

☐ Unsure   ☐ Tends not to be true

☐ Definitely not true

➤ My Christian faith is an important source of strength and comfort in my life.

☐ Definitely true of me   ☐ Tends to be true

☐ Unsure   ☐ Tends not to be true

☐ Definitely not true

Other important questions to ask yourself:

> Do I understand that good health requires balance in all areas of my life?

> Am I willing to open myself up to the spiritual support of others?

> How does my faith influence my daily habits and choices?

A strong faith and regular prayer do not guarantee you will live a long life or be free from disease; they simply lower your risk. It's important to know that emotional stress and physical illness are not forms of divine punishment. God loves you and desires the very best for you (see Romans 8:31-32). However, your daily choices can have a strong influence on your overall health and well-being. Your personal faith can be a strong motivator for healthy and purposeful living.

STOCKING THE HEALTHY KITCHEN

Deciding to eat more healthfully is easy. It's much more difficult to actually make it happen! This can be particularly challenging for meals prepared at home. How many times have your intentions been good, but there just wasn't anything good to fix for dinner? If healthy food choices aren't kept in the kitchen, then the battle is lost before it's begun.

It is essential that your kitchen shelves reflect the new food goals you have set for yourself. Does this mean purchasing all fat-free, sugar-free and no-taste foods? Of course not! It does mean keeping certain foods on hand to provide you with lots of healthy choices. There are several things to consider as you begin planning your healthy kitchen.

FOODS YOU WILL REALLY EAT

Don't purchase foods because you *think* you should eat them. Purchase foods you *know* you'll eat. If rice cakes don't really suit your taste buds, don't buy them. Low-fat animal crackers or graham crackers may be more to your liking—keep these on hand instead. You'll have to experiment a little to find what healthy foods you like best.

FREQUENCY OF USE

This is particularly important for cooking oils, flours, snack items, meat, and fresh fruits and vegetables. Some foods, such as olive oil, might be used in small amounts. Buying in smaller quantities allows for greater freshness and less waste. Some foods tend to dry out and become stale quickly. It is better to buy single-serving sizes and enjoy all of them than to eat a few and throw out the rest. Using canned and frozen fruits and vegetables are great choices, especially if you find your fresh versions are spoiling before you eat them. Freezing breads and flours is a good way to preserve their freshness.

Preparation Time

For most people, time is a big consideration when planning a meal. Having a refrigerator stocked full of fresh produce and lean meat looks great, but if there isn't time to cook, it usually just ends up in the trash. Anticipate having a few times when you won't have time to cook. Keep some low-fat convenience foods on hand so that you're not caught unprepared. Cooking extra and freezing the leftovers in single servings is a great way to have your own fast food!

After seriously considering your needs and preferences, go ahead and make out a kitchen list. Start by making a list of what you *normally* buy— no special foods or changes. Review your list to see if there are some items that you're willing to make healthy substitutions for. For example, you may be willing to trade nonfat milk for 2 percent milk. Maybe the fried tortilla chips could be traded for baked chips or pretzels. You should also make a list of new foods you're willing to try. Of course, this is not an exhaustive list, but it should get you headed in the right direction. With time you will discover the items you need in your kitchen for healthy eating. The trick is to stock a kitchen that works best for you and provides a variety of healthy foods to choose from anytime.

Basic Items to Keep on Hand

This is not an exhaustive list, but it should get you headed in the right direction. With time you will discover the items you need in your kitchen for healthy eating. The trick is to stock a kitchen that works best for you and provides a variety of healthy foods to choose from anytime.

In the Freezer

Frozen vegetables	Buy in bags instead of boxes; it allows you to use only what you need. You can buy individual servings too.
Frozen entrées	Choose entrées with 200 to 300 calories, 10 or fewer grams of fat and 400 or fewer milligrams of sodium.
Snacks	Choose low-calorie items, such as fruit bars or sherbet.

In the Refrigerator

Eggs	Eggs are a great source of lean protein, as well as a common ingredient for most baking. Learn to cook with egg whites and leave the yolk behind. Egg substitutes are also fine.
Milk	Keep plenty of low-fat or nonfat milk on hand (1 percent or lower); it's a great source of calcium.
Cheese	Reduced-fat or low-fat cheeses are your best choices. When you only have time for quick meal, a slice of cheese with whole-grain bread is a healthy choice. Grated cheese allows you to use less for the same amount of flavor; choose sharp flavors.
Lunch meats	Keep a low-fat variety on hand, such as turkey or chicken breast. Be sure to purchase in quantities that you actually eat! Try to choose low-sodium versions.
Salad in a bag	It's washed and ready to go! Use nonfat or low-fat dressing.
Salad dressing	Choose light, low-fat, reduced-fat, nonfat or low-calorie varieties; you may have to experiment to find one or two favorites.
Fruits and vegetables	Make a list of your favorites and stock up every time you go to the store. Buy only what you can eat in one week. Cut up your vegetables when you first get home from the store, so they're ready to go. Juices are also a good choice when you're on the run.

In the Pantry

Oils	Choose at least one monounsaturated oil (olive or canola) and one polyunsaturated oil (corn, safflower or sunflower). Purchase the amount you'll use within a few months, so that it doesn't go bad before you get to it.
Nonstick spray	Essential for low-fat cooking. Specialty stores sell spray bottles, so that you can make your own.
Canned foods	Keep canned vegetables such as corn, green beans, canned tomatoes, etc. These are commonly used items in casseroles and soups. Look for low-sodium varieties.
Pasta	Always have a package of pasta on hand! Choose a prepared pasta sauce that's low in fat. Prepackaged pasta dishes can be high in fat and sodium.
Rice	Add rice to a variety of meals. You may want to have two or three varieties, such as wild rice, basmati and your favorite flavored rice (watch out for sodium).
Cereal	Keep plenty of low-fat cereal around. Good choices are shredded wheat, bran cereals and oatmeal.
Other breakfast foods	Low-fat pop tarts or granola bars for those grab-n-go mornings
Snacks	Choose only healthy snack foods: popcorn, low-fat cookies, low-fat snack crackers, rice cakes, dried fruits, etc. You can't eat what's not in the house!
Herbs and spices	Make sure you have lots of herbs and spices on hand. Don't be afraid to try new ones! Keep a list of your favorites; replace them after about one year. *Hint: Write the date of purchase on the container with a permanent-ink felt pen.*

STRATEGIES FOR SOCIAL SITUATIONS

Special occasions are usually wonderful times for fellowship and enjoying good food. Unfortunately, too much of the focus is on too much food and foods too high in calories, fat and sugar! Are there certain situations that cause you to give up or give in? It's not uncommon for the holidays or a special get-together to derail your healthy eating plan. Does this mean you can't have any fun at the party? Of course not! What it means is that you need to anticipate the challenges and make a plan to stick with your healthy goals. Planning ahead is the key to success!

Will the satisfaction you get by sticking with your goal for healthy eating outweigh any pleasure you might get from overeating or choosing foods high in calories, fat and sugar?

TIPS FOR SUCCESS ON ANY OCCASION

The next time you are attending a party or special get-together, remember some basic rules for success.

Anticipate Difficult Situations

Before going to the party, picture in your mind how the event will go. What kinds of foods will be there? Anticipate situations and food temptations that will be difficult for you. Imagine yourself being in control of your eating and making healthy choices. Set some ground rules for yourself before you get there:

- Decide to fill your plate only one time.
- Limit yourself to small servings.
- Eat before you go, and enjoy the fellowship instead; never go to a special event hungry.
- Make up your mind to avoid the tempting high-fat, high-calorie choices.
- Ask someone to hold you accountable.
- Decide in advance that you'll only eat a few bites of your favorite food.

- Check out the available foods, and choose only one or two that are your *absolute* favorites and leave the rest behind.
- If it is a potluck event, bring a delicious low-fat version of a favorite. It just might be the hit of the party!
- Eat slowly; it takes about 20 minutes for your brain to get the message that your stomach is full.

Keep Burning the Calories

On the day (or for a day or two after) of a special occasion, make sure you fit in your physical activity. Taking a brisk walk prior to the event can help curb your appetite. Just participating in exercise helps to boost motivation and provides encouragement for managing tempting situations. Physical activity is also a great way to burn calories. You may have to exercise in the morning or at other times to guarantee you'll fit it in. Be creative and fit in physical activity however you can.

Focus on Fun and Fellowship

The relationships you build and the fun times will be much more valuable to you than any of the foods you might eat. Decide ahead of time that you'll have a meaningful conversation with several people at the gathering. Focus on others, rather than on yourself and your appetite. In fact, nutrition and health might be a good topic of conversation. Let others know what you're doing in First Place—a little lifestyle evangelism! Don't visit with others while standing next to the food, and try not to eat while talking with other people; hold a low-calorie beverage in your hand instead.

➺ What strategies are you ready to try, so you can experience success no matter what the occasion?

Success Tips for Specific Occasions

Business and Meetings

If you're in the business world, you may attend seminars, meetings and other special events. You may also have to travel. If you're not in the business world, you probably attend a lot of meetings anyway: church meetings, Bible study, community meetings and get-togethers with family and friends. Unfortunately, most of these occasions involve food. By planning ahead you can stick with your goals for a healthy lifestyle.

- Decide ahead of time to pack your own snacks: raw vegetables, fruit, low-fat crackers, pretzels or a whole-grain bagel.

- Bringing your own snack will provide you with a backup in case no healthy foods are offered. It's also a great way to curb your appetite if a meeting runs long.

- Make sure you drink plenty of water. Avoid high-calorie beverages, such as soft drinks and coffee with cream.

- Make time for physical activity. Sitting for hours at a time can cause boredom, which triggers snacking. Even a 5- or 10-minute walk is helpful.

- Watch out for buffet-style food service. Load up on fresh fruits, vegetables and other low-fat choices. Don't load your plate just because "it's all you can eat." Rather than trying all the foods, pick one or two of your favorites and keep your portions small.

- If you're providing the food or bringing a dish, make sure it's healthy. Don't feel you have to please people with high-fat desserts and other foods. You'll be surprised at how appreciative people will be at your thoughtfulness.

Holidays and Parties

Special occasions are celebrated with special foods! During these times, tempting foods are usually everywhere, and everyone is eating them and offering them to you. What situations are most difficult for you? With some simple strategies, holidays and parties can be enjoyed without the guilt of overdoing it. Here are some strategies to help get you started.

- Prepare in advance for holidays and parties. Make a commitment to stick with your goals.

- Stick to your regular eating schedule. This will help you avoid the all-day grazing that can sometimes occur when food is always around.

- Remember to eat slowly and concentrate on enjoying the foods you eat.

- Because special foods are always around, taste small portions of the items that are truly unique to the season and leave the everyday foods alone.

- Rather than overdoing it every day, plan for one or two special meals you'll really enjoy; make up for these by eating healthy the rest of the time.

- Learn to say "No, thank you." It's okay to turn down food politely. Have a plan for what you'll say.

- Make sure you take time to relax before and during special occasions and during holidays. Spend some time praying and meditating about ways that will help you stick with your goals.

- Don't allow yourself to gain weight over the holidays; weigh yourself at least once a week. Cut back and resume your eating plan if you notice your weight creeping upward.

- Plan enjoyable activities that are not centered around food; be creative.

- If you're the host, plan to serve healthy foods. Learn to make low-fat substitutions in the recipes for some of your favorite holiday foods.

- Avoid all-or-nothing thinking; don't deprive yourself or feel guilty about enjoying certain foods. The secret to healthy eating for special occasions is to have a plan and remember the principles of balance, moderation and variety.

UNDERSTANDING HIGH BLOOD PRESSURE

Fifty million—nearly one out of four—Americans have high blood pressure. More than half of all Americans over the age of 65 have high blood pressure! Unfortunately, many people are not aware they have it. High blood pressure is often called the silent killer because it usually causes no symptoms. If your blood pressure is high, you're at a much greater risk for heart attack, stroke and kidney disease. It's important to know your blood pressure and take steps to bring it down if it's high. A healthy lifestyle can lower your risk of developing high blood pressure in the future.

WHAT IS BLOOD PRESSURE?

You've probably had your blood pressure measured before, but you may not know what the two numbers mean. The numbers tell you how hard your blood is pressing on the walls of your arteries as it flows through your body. If your blood pressure is high, your heart and arteries are working too hard. High blood pressure can damage the heart, arteries and organs such as the brain and kidneys. The first or top number is the systolic pressure. This is the pressure created in the arteries when the heart contracts. The second or bottom number is the diastolic pressure. This is the pressure in the arteries when the heart relaxes between beats. What are your blood-pressure numbers?

Risk Classification	Systolic (mmHg)	Diastolic (mmHg)	My Blood Pressure
Optimal	120	80	
Normal	120 to 139	80 to 84	
High Normal	130 to 139	85 to 89	
High	140	90	

If your blood pressure is 140/90 or greater, talk to your doctor and begin making healthful lifestyle changes today. If you're in the high normal range, watch your blood pressure very closely. If you don't know your blood pressure, get it measured. No matter what your blood pressure, a healthy lifestyle can help you keep it low.

CAUSES OF HIGH BLOOD PRESSURE

Doctors don't know all the factors that cause high blood pressure. In at least 90 percent of people the cause is unknown. In such cases, the diagnosis is called "primary," or "essential," hypertension. High blood pressure often runs in families and the risk increases with age. Several lifestyle factors also seem to be associated with high blood pressure: weight gain and obesity, a sedentary lifestyle and poor dietary habits.

PREVENTION OF HIGH BLOOD PRESSURE

Fortunately, a healthy lifestyle can lower your chances of developing high blood pressure or help lower it if it's already high. Doctors now recommend "the big five" lifestyle strategies to control blood pressure.

1. Achieve and maintain a healthy weight.
2. Get and stay physically active.
3. Follow an eating plan high in fruits, vegetables and low-fat dairy foods.
4. Cut down on sodium.
5. Limit or eliminate alcohol.

ACHIEVE AND MAINTAIN A HEALTHY WEIGHT

As your body weight rises, blood pressure often rises too. If you are overweight, losing as little as 10 percent of your weight can significantly decrease your risk of developing high blood pressure or lower it if it's high. Losing weight can also lower your risk for heart attack, stroke and diabetes. Monitor your blood pressure every few months as you lose weight.

Get and Stay Physically Active

Regular, moderate physical activity can lower your blood pressure and improve your health and well-being. Try to do at least 30 minutes of activity on most, preferably all, days of the week. Brisk walking, gardening, bicycling and swimming are good examples of moderate activities. Pick activities that you enjoy and make them a part of your everyday life. Select an activity that requires some exertion but is comfortable and enjoyable. Continue this activity on a regular basis; when it becomes less challenging, gradually increase the time or intensity or add another activity you enjoy. You don't have to do 30 minutes at one time. You can break it into sessions of 10 to 15 minutes two or three times a day. This may help you get started.

Follow a Healthy Eating Plan

For years, doctors have known the benefits of cutting down on sodium and alcohol intake. In fact, studies show that the combination of modest weight loss and limited sodium intake can reverse high blood pressure in many people. The latest news on controlling blood pressure, however, comes from a study called DASH—Dietary Approaches to Stop Hypertension. The DASH study found that eating the right foods can lower blood pressure as effectively as taking medication.

The DASH Diet

- High in fruits and vegetables—7 to 10 servings daily.
- High in low-fat dairy foods—2 to 3 servings daily.
- High in grains (breads, cereal, rice and pasta)—6 or more servings daily.
- Moderate amounts of lean meat, chicken or fish daily—no more than 2 servings daily.
- Legumes, nuts and seeds—4 to 5 servings weekly (more beans than nuts or seeds).
- Low in fat and saturated fat—no more than 2 to 3 daily servings of fats, such as oils, margarine, mayonnaise or salad dressing.

- Low in sweets—no more than 5 low-fat sweets each week. Fruit is the preferred dessert.
- The DASH study did not involve efforts to lose weight or restrict sodium.

The DASH researchers don't understand all the reasons that this eating plan is so beneficial. One reason may be its high potassium, magnesium and calcium content.

There is good evidence that salt restriction can lower blood pressure. Higher salt intake is related to higher blood pressure in some people. Cutting back on salt and sodium may help keep blood pressure low. Use less salt in cooking and at the table. Most salt and sodium come from processed and fast foods. Learn to read labels and buy low-salt alternatives.

Reducing alcohol intake can also lower blood pressure. In addition to increasing blood pressure, excessive alcohol consumption can cause a variety of other serious health problems, such as liver, kidney or heart disease.

≫ What steps do you need to take to insure a healthy blood pressure level?

FIRST PLACE
MENU PLANS

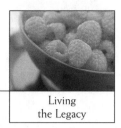

Living
the Legacy

Each plan is based on approximately 1,400 calories.

Breakfast   2 breads, 1 fruit, 1 milk, 0-½ fat
(When a meat exchange is used, milk is omitted.)

Lunch   2 meats, 2 breads, 1 vegetable, 1 fruit, 1 fat

Dinner   3 meats, 2 breads, 2 vegetables, 1 fat

Snacks   1 bread, 1 fruit, 1 milk, ½-1 fat (or any remaining exchanges)

For more calories, add the following to the 1,400 calorie plan.

1,600 calories   2 breads, 1 fat

1,800 calories   2 meats, 3 breads, 1 vegetable, 1 fat

2,000 calories   2 meats, 4 breads, 1 vegetable, 3 fats

2,200 calories   2 meats, 5 breads, 1 vegetable, 1 fruit, 5 fats

2,400 calories   2 meats, 6 breads, 2 vegetables, 1 fruit, 6 fats

The exchanges for these meals were calculated using the MasterCook software. It uses a database of over 6,000 food items prepared using United States Department of Agriculture (USDA) publications and information from food manufacturers. As with any nutritional program, MasterCook calculates the nutritional values of the recipes based on ingredients. Nutrition may vary due to how the food is prepared, where the food comes from, i.e., geography, soil content, season, ripeness, processing and method of preparation. For these reasons, please use the recipes and menu plans as approximate guides. As always consult your physician and/or a registered dietician before starting a diet program.

🍎 Breakfast

1 c. bran-flakes cereal
½ medium papaya
1 c. nonfat milk

Exchanges: 2 breads, 1 fruit, 1 milk

~~~~~~

2 slices diet whole-wheat bread, toasted
1 tbsp. reduced-fat peanut butter
½ medium grapefruit
1 c. nonfat milk

Exchanges: ½ meat, 1 bread, ½ fruit, 1 milk, ½ fat

~~~~~~

2 low-fat frozen waffles, heated
1 tsp. reduced-calorie margarine
2 tsp. sugar-free syrup
½ small mango
1 c. nonfat milk

Exchanges: 2 breads, 1 fruit, 1 milk, ½ fat

~~~~~~

Raisin French Toast

1½ slices cinnamon-raisin bread
¼ c. egg substitute
¼ tsp. vanilla flavoring
1 tbsp. nonfat milk
   Nonstick cooking spray

In a shallow bowl, combine egg substitute, vanilla and milk; add slices of bread, turning until egg mixture is absorbed. Spray a small nonstick skillet or griddle with nonstick cooking spray; preheat. Cook bread over medium heat 3 to 5 minutes, turning once, until golden brown on both sides.

Serve with 1 tablespoon sugar-free syrup, ½ cup grapefruit sections and ½ cup nonfat milk.

Exchanges: ½ meat, 2 breads, ½ fruit, ½ milk

1   small (2 oz.) diet bran muffin

1   tsp. reduced-calorie margarine

1   tsp. peach jam

½   medium banana

1   c. plain nonfat yogurt

Exchanges: 2 breads, 1 fruit, 1 milk, ½ fat

~~~~~~

1 ½   c. puffed-wheat cereal

1   large tangerine

1   c. nonfat milk

Exchanges: 2 breads, 1 fruit, 1 milk

~~~~~~

½   c. cornflakes cereal

2   slices diet whole-wheat bread, toasted

1   tbsp. fat-free cream cheese

½   c. sliced strawberries

1   c. nonfat milk

Exchanges: ½ meat, 2 breads, ½ fruit, 1 milk

~~~~~~

2   frozen pancakes, heated

1   tbsp. sugar-free syrup

1   tsp. reduced-calorie margarine

    2-in. wedge honeydew melon

1   c. nonfat milk

Exchanges: 2 breads, 1 fruit, 1 milk, ½ fat

~~~~~~

1   small (2 oz.) whole-wheat English muffin, split and toasted

1   tsp. reduced-calorie margarine

1   c. sliced strawberries

½   c. nonfat milk

Exchanges: 2 breads, 1 fruit, 1 milk, ½ fat

~~~~~~

2   slices cinnamon-raisin bread, toasted

1   tsp. reduced-calorie margarine

½   tsp. granulated sugar

    Pinch cinnamon

¾   c. plain nonfat yogurt

¾   c. blueberries

Exchanges: 2 breads, 1 fruit, 1 milk, ½ fat

½   c. cornflakes cereal

2   slices diet whole-wheat bread, toasted

1   tsp. reduced-calorie margarine

½   medium banana, sliced

½   c. nonfat milk

Exchanges: 2 breads, 1 fruit, ½ milk, ½ fat

~~~~~~

2   slices diet sourdough bread, toasted

1   tsp. reduced-calorie margarine

¾   c. blueberries

1   c. nonfat milk

Exchanges: 2 breads, 1 fruit, 1 milk, ½ fat

~~~~~~

1½   c. fortified-flakes cereal

½   small mango

1   c. nonfat milk

Exchanges: 2 breads, 1 fruit, 1 milk

~~~~~~

1   small (2 oz.) bagel

1   tsp. strawberry jam

1   c. artificially sweetened mixed-berry nonfat yogurt

¾   c. blackberries

Exchanges: 2 breads, 1 fruit, 1 milk

~~~~~~

❧ LUNCH

Pastrami Sandwich

2   slices diet rye bread

2   oz. cooked turkey pastrami, sliced

1   tsp. prepared spicy brown mustard

1   tsp. low-fat mayonnaise

2   tomato slices

¼   c. alfalfa sprouts

2   romaine lettuce leaves

Serve with ¼ cup coleslaw, ½ cup each cucumber sticks and whole radishes, and ½ cup tropical fruit salad.

Exchanges: 2 meats, 1 bread, 2 vegetables, 1 fruit, 1 fat

Spinach-and-Cheddar-Stuffed Potato

1   6-oz. baked potato
1   tsp. reduced-calorie margarine
½   c. cooked chopped spinach
1½ oz. reduced-fat cheddar cheese, grated

Cut a lengthwise slit about 1-inch deep into potato, cutting to within ½-inch of each end; gently squeeze ends together until potato opens. Top potato pulp with margarine, add spinach and cheddar cheese; microwave on high (100 percent power) for 1½ to 2 minutes or until heated through.

Serve with 1 cup each carrot and celery sticks.
Exchanges: ½ **meat, 2 breads, 2 vegetables, 1 fat**

~~~~~~

1   slice thin-crust cheese pizza
2   c. torn green leaf or romaine lettuce
½   c. cooked artichoke hearts, chilled
2   oz. cooked chickpeas, drained
½   c. carrots
½   c. zucchini sticks
2   tbsp. low-fat Italian dressing
1   small apple

Exchanges: 2 meats, 2 breads, 2 vegetables, 1 fruit, 1½ fats

~~~~~~

Honey-Roasted Turkey Sandwich

1   whole-wheat pita, split in half to form 2 pockets
1   tsp. low-fat mayonnaise
2   oz. honey-roasted turkey, thinly sliced
2   tomato slices
1   romaine lettuce leaf

Slice pita in half crosswise; open to form 2 pockets. Assemble sandwich.

Serve with ½ cup each red bell pepper strips and zucchini sticks, and 1 small pear.
Exchanges: 2 meats, 2 breads, 1 vegetable, 1 fruit, ½ fat

~~~~~~

Smoked Chicken Sandwich

2 slices diet multigrain bread
2 oz. smoked boneless, skinless chicken breast, thinly sliced

2 tsp. low-fat mayonnaise
¼ c. alfalfa sprouts
2 romaine lettuce leaves

Serve with ½ cup carrot sticks, 1 cup artificially sweetened black-cherry nonfat yogurt and **Cucumber Salad**. (In small bowl, combine ½ cup cucumber slices, 1 teaspoon each vegetable oil and rice wine vinegar, and pinch ground white pepper.)
Exchanges: 2 meats, 1 bread, 2 vegetables, 1 milk

~~~~~~

Chicken Sandwich

2 slices diet rye bread
2 oz. cooked boneless, skinless chicken breast, sliced
1 tbsp. fat-free Thousand Island dressing

2 tomato slices
¼ c. shredded romaine lettuce

Serve with 1 small apple and ½ cup each carrot and zucchini sticks with 2 tablespoons low-fat ranch dressing.
Exchanges: 2 meats, 1 bread, 1 vegetable, 1 fruit, ½ fat

~~~~~~

BBQ Chicken Salad

10 oz. boneless, skinless chicken breasts
2 tsp. mild or hot chili powder
2 tsp. onion powder
1 tsp. garlic powder
1 tsp. paprika
8 c. torn romaine lettuce leaves

2 medium tomatoes, each sliced into 8 wedges
1 c. cooked corn
2 thin red onion slices, separated into rings
2 tbsp. low-fat ranch dressing

Preheat oven to 350° F. In small bowl, combine chili powder, onion powder, garlic powder and paprika; rub mixture evenly over both sides of chicken breasts. Place chicken onto large sheet of foil; wrap tightly, crimping edges to seal. Place foil packet onto baking sheet; bake 8 to 10 minutes. Carefully open packet; bake 6 to 8 minutes more or until chicken is cooked through and juices run clear when pierced with fork. Set aside to cool.

While chicken is cooling, line large bowl with lettuce; top with tomatoes, corn and onion. Shred cooled chicken with fork; add to lettuce mixture. Drizzle evenly with dressing. Serves 4.

Serve with 1 cup broccoli florets, a 1-ounce whole-wheat roll with 1 teaspoon reduced-calorie margarine, and 1 medium peach.

Exchanges: 2 meats, 2 breads, 1 vegetable, 1 fruit, ½ fat

Boston Market Open-Faced Turkey Club Sandwich

(No cheese or sauce)

    1 c. carrot sticks
    2 tbsp. low-fat ranch dressing
    1 c. fruit salad

Exchanges: 2 meats, 2 breads, 1 vegetable, 1 fruit, ½ fat

Oriental Seafood Pasta Salad

    2 oz. (about 6 medium) cooked   ½ c. sliced celery
       shrimp, peeled and deveined   ¼ c. cooked red kidney beans,
    ½ c. cooked rotini pasta   drained
    ½ c. bean sprouts   ½ c. mandarin oranges

Dressing

    1 tbsp. rice wine vinegar
    ½ tsp. oriental sesame oil

Combine all ingredients in medium bowl; toss with dressing.

Serve with ½ toasted pita bread.

Exchanges: 1 meat, 3 breads, 1 vegetable, 1 fruit, ½ fat

Roast Beef Sandwich

    1 6-in. whole-wheat pita   1 tsp. prepared mustard
    2 oz. cooked, lean, boneless   2 tomato slices
       roast beef, thinly sliced   1 romaine lettuce leaf
    1 tsp. low-fat mayonnaise

Cut pita in half crosswise; open to form 2 pockets. Assemble sandwich.

Serve with ½ cup each carrot and cucumber sticks.

Exchanges: 2 meats, 2 breads, 1 vegetable, ½ fat

Turkey Sandwich

2 slices diet rye bread

2 oz. roasted boneless, skinless turkey breast, sliced

1 tsp. low-fat mayonnaise

1 tsp. prepared mustard

½ medium tomato, sliced

½ c. romaine or spinach leaves

Serve with ½ cup each red and green bell pepper strips and 1 cup artificially sweetened coffee-flavored nonfat yogurt.

Exchanges: 2 meats, 1 bread, 1 vegetable, 1 milk, ½ fat

Healthy Choice Pepper Steak Entrée (11 oz.)

1 c. green salad

2 tbsp. low-fat dressing

½ c. fruit salad

Exchanges: 2 meats, 2 breads, 1 vegetable, 1 fruit

Chef Salad

¾ oz. cooked turkey, diced

¾ oz. cooked ham, diced

1½ c. mixed salad greens (dark green)

1 c. combined chopped broccoli, zucchini, carrots, onion, cauliflower and bell pepper

¾ oz. reduced-fat Swiss cheese, diced

2 tbsp. reduced-fat dressing

⅓ c. mandarin oranges

Serve with 8 saltine crackers.

Exchanges: 2 meats, 1 bread, 1 vegetable, 1 fruit, 1 fat

Soup and Salad

1 serving Campbell's Chunky Sirloin Burger Soup

1 small (1 oz.) breadstick

1 oz. reduced-fat Colby-Jack cheese, grated

2 plums

Exchanges: 2 meats, 2½ breads, 1 vegetable, ½ fat, 1 fruit

Chicken Biscuit Stew

4	3-oz. boneless, skinless chicken breasts, cooked and cubed
2	tbsp. reduced-calorie margarine
½	c. all-purpose flour
¼	tsp. salt
¼	tsp. pepper
½	c. nonfat milk
1	10½-oz. can chicken broth
⅓	c. chopped onion
1	8½-oz. can cut green beans, drained
1	8¼-oz. can sliced carrots, drained
1	4½-oz. can refrigerated buttermilk biscuits

Preheat oven to 375° F. In heavy saucepan, melt margarine over medium-high heat; stir in flour, salt and pepper. Gradually add milk and broth, stirring with a whisk until blended. Cook 4 minutes or until thick and bubbly, stirring constantly. Add chicken, onion, green beans and carrots; cook 1 minute and remove from heat. Carefully split biscuits in half horizontally; place over chicken mixture to create topping. Bake 20 minutes or until biscuits are golden brown. Serves 4.

Exchanges: 2½ meats, 2 breads, 1 vegetable, 1½ fats

~ ~

Chicken Pita Sandwiches

1	lb. boneless, skinless chicken breasts
⅓	c. fresh lemon juice
¾	tsp. olive oil
1½	garlic cloves, minced
½	tsp. curry powder
	Dash salt and pepper
1	c. thinly sliced cucumber
½	c. thinly sliced onion, separated into rings
1½	tsp. minced fresh mint
½	8-oz. carton plain low-fat yogurt
4	6-in. whole-wheat pita bread rounds, cut in half
½	c. thinly sliced romaine lettuce
½	c. chopped tomato
	Nonstick cooking spray

THE DAY BEFORE, place chicken breasts, lemon juice, oil, garlic, curry and salt and pepper in large zip-top plastic bag; seal and shake well to coat chicken. Marinate in refrigerator overnight, turning bag occasionally.

NEXT DAY, combine cucumber, onion, mint and yogurt in a bowl; stir well. Cover and chill. Spray BBQ grill rack with cooking spray; preheat grill. Remove chicken from bag, reserving marinade. Grill chicken 10 minutes each side or until done, basting occasionally with reserved marinade. Let cool. Cut diagonally across grain into $\frac{1}{4}$-inch slices; set aside. Spoon 1 tablespoon lettuce, 1 tablespoon tomato and 1$\frac{1}{2}$ tablespoons yogurt sauce into each pita half; top with chicken. Serves 4.

Serve each with $\frac{1}{2}$ cup carrot sticks and 2 tablespoons low-fat ranch dressing.

Exchanges: 3 meats, 2$\frac{1}{2}$ breads, 1 vegetable, 1 fat

~~~~~~

Citrus Shrimp Salad

1 lb. medium shrimp, uncooked and unpeeled	2$\frac{1}{4}$ tsp. Dijon mustard
1 qt. water	1$\frac{1}{2}$ tsp. honey
1 tbsp. seasoned salt	Dash pepper
2 tbsp. low-fat Italian dressing	2 c. sliced romaine lettuce
1$\frac{1}{2}$ tbsp. finely chopped shallots	1 c. pink grapefruit sections
1 tbsp. red wine vinegar	(about 4 large grapefruit)
1 tbsp. plain nonfat yogurt	1 c. orange sections
1 tbsp. orange juice	(about 5 oranges)
2 tbsp. chopped fresh chives	

Bring water and seasoned salt to a boil; add shrimp. Cook 3 to 5 minutes; drain and rinse with cold water. Peel and devein shrimp; chill. In large bowl, combine dressing, shallots, vinegar, yogurt, orange juice, mustard, honey and pepper; mix well. Add shrimp and stir to coat. Line large platter with lettuce; spoon shrimp mixture into center of platter; arrange grapefruit sections and orange sections around salad. Garnish with chives. Serves 4.

Serve with 5 slices melba toast.

Exchanges: 2 meats, 1 bread, $\frac{1}{2}$ vegetable, $\frac{1}{2}$ fruit

~~~~~~

Chicken and Broccoli Frittata

1 ½ c. chopped roasted chicken
2 c. chopped broccoli florets
2 tbsp. dry bread crumbs
3 tbsp. all-purpose flour
1 tsp. dried basil
¼ tsp. salt
⅛ tsp. pepper
Nonstick cooking spray

1 c. nonfat milk
1 tsp. Dijon mustard
1 4-oz. carton egg substitute
½ c. shredded, reduced-fat, extra-sharp cheddar cheese, divided
¼ tsp. paprika

~~~~~~

Preheat oven to 350° F. Cook broccoli in boiling water 3 minutes or until tender-crisp. Drain and set aside. Coat 9-inch pie pan with cooking spray; sprinkle with bread crumbs (do not remove excess crumbs); set aside. In large bowl, combine flour, basil, salt and pepper; add milk and mustard. Blend well with whisk; stir in egg substitute. Add chicken and ¼ cup cheese; stir well. Pour mixture into pie pan; sprinkle with remaining cheese and paprika. Bake 45 minutes or until set. Let cool on rack 5 minutes before slicing. Serves 4.

Serve each with a 1-ounce dinner roll, 1 cup green salad with 2 tablespoons low-fat dressing.
Exchanges: 3 meats, 1 ½ breads, 1 vegetable, 1 fat

~~~~~~

Indonesian Snapper Fillets

4 4-oz. snapper fillets, about 1 in. thick
¼ c. fresh lemon juice
1 tbsp. curry powder
1 tbsp. sesame oil

1 8-oz. carton plain nonfat yogurt
¼ tsp. salt
⅛ tsp. pepper
Nonstick cooking spray

Coat broiler rack with cooking spray; preheat broiler. Combine lemon juice, curry, sesame oil and yogurt in large zip-top plastic bag. Add fillets; seal and marinate in refrigerator 20 minutes. Remove fillets from bag and discard marinade. Arrange fillets on broiler rack; sprinkle with salt and pepper. Broil 8 minutes or until fillets flake easily with fork. Serves 4.

Serve each with ½ cup sautéed snap peas and 1 cup cooked linguine tossed with 2 teaspoons teriyaki sauce.
Exchanges: 3 meats, 2 breads, 1 vegetable, ¼ milk, 1 ½ fats

~~~~~~

Ginger Salmon Fillets

4　4-oz. salmon fillets,
　　about 1 in. thick
¼　c. fresh orange juice
¼　c. soy sauce
¼　c. cooking sherry
¼　c. Dijon mustard

2　tbsp. grated peeled fresh ginger
2　tbsp. honey
　　Green onion fans* (optional)
　　Nonstick cooking spray

*Here's how to make a green-onion fan: Cut off the root of a green onion and then slice into the white end 2 or 3 times to create thin strips. Place in cold water for 1 hour and the onion will "fan"!

Coat broiler rack with cooking spray; preheat broiler. Combine orange juice, soy sauce, cooking sherry, ginger and honey in large zip-top plastic bag. Add fillets; seal and marinate in refrigerator 30 minutes. Remove fillets from bag and reserve marinade. Arrange fillets on broiler rack; sprinkle with salt and pepper. Broil 6 minutes or until fillets flake easily with fork, basting frequently with reserved marinade. After fillets are cooked, place remaining marinade in saucepan; bring to a boil and use as a sauce for serving. Garnish with green-onion fans, if desired. Serves 4.

Serve each with ⅔ cup roasted potatoes, 1 cup cooked green vegetables and a 1-ounce dinner roll topped with 1 teaspoon reduced-fat margarine.
Exchanges: 3 meats, 2 breads, 2 vegetables, ½ fat

~ ~

Chicken and Fettuccine

1　lb. boneless, skinless chicken
　　breasts, cut into 1-in. pieces
2　tsp. vegetable oil
1½　c. sliced mushrooms
½　c. chopped onion
1　garlic clove, minced
½ tsp. salt

½　tsp. dried basil
¼　tsp. pepper
2　c. coarsely chopped tomato
4　c. hot cooked fettuccine
　　(about 8 oz. uncooked)
¼　c. freshly grated Parmesan
　　cheese

Heat oil in large nonstick skillet over medium-high heat. Add mushrooms, onion and garlic; sauté 2 minutes. Add chicken, salt, basil and pepper; sauté 5 minutes more or until chicken is cooked through. Add tomato; sauté 2 minutes more. Serve over pasta; sprinkle with cheese. Serves 4.

Serve each with 1 cup green salad with 2 tablespoons low-fat dressing.
Exchanges: 3 meats, 2½ breads, 1½ vegetables, 1 fat

~ ~

Hearty Vegetable and Beef Stew

¾ lb. boneless, lean chuck roast, trimmed of fat and cut into ½-in. cubes

2 14 ¼-oz. cans fat-free beef broth

2 tsp. olive oil, divided

1 large onion, sliced

⅓ c. tomato paste

3 garlic cloves, minced

3 c. cubed carrots

3 c. cubed red potatoes

2½ c. quartered mushrooms

½ c. red cooking wine

¼ tsp. pepper

1 8-oz. can cut green beans

2 tbsp. water

1 tbsp. cornstarch

Chopped fresh parsley (optional)

In medium saucepan, bring beef broth to boil. Cook 15 minutes or until reduced to 2 cups; remove from heat and set aside. In large Dutch oven, heat 1 teaspoon oil over medium-high heat. Add beef; brown on one side and remove from pan. Heat remaining oil in pan over medium-high heat; add onion, tomato paste and garlic; cook 5 minutes, stirring constantly. Return beef to pan; add reduced broth, carrots, potatoes, mushrooms, cooking wine, pepper and green beans. Bring to boil; cover, reduce heat and simmer 45 minutes or until vegetables are tender. In small bowl, combine water and cornstarch; stir well to remove lumps. Add to stew; bring to a boil and cook 1 minute, stirring constantly. Ladle 2 cups of stew into each soup bowl; garnish with parsley, if desired. Serves 4.

Serve each with 1 cup salad with 2 tablespoons low-fat dressing.
Exchanges: 2 meats, 2 breads, 2 vegetables, 1 fat

~~~~~~

Cheese-and-Hamburger Casserole

½ lb. lean (15% or less fat) ground beef

½ c. chopped onion

1½ garlic cloves, crushed

4 oz. sliced mushrooms

½ c. spaghetti sauce

Dash pepper

½ 28-oz. can whole tomatoes, undrained and chopped

2½ tbsp. all-purpose flour

1¼ c. nonfat evaporated milk

½ c. crumbled feta cheese

½ c. shredded part-skim mozzarella cheese

2 c. uncooked penne pasta

1½ tsp. chopped fresh parsley (optional)

THE DAY BEFORE, combine ground beef, onion and garlic in large nonstick skillet; cook over medium-high heat until browned, stirring to crumble meat. Add mushrooms; cook 5 minutes more or until tender. Add spaghetti sauce, pepper and tomatoes; stir well. Bring to a boil; reduce heat and simmer uncovered for 20 minutes. Set aside. Place flour in medium saucepan. Gradually add milk, stirring with a whisk until blended. Cook over medium heat 10 minutes or until thick, stirring constantly. Stir in cheeses; cook 3 minutes or until cheeses melt, stirring constantly. Reserve ½ cup cheese sauce; pour remainder along with beef mixture and pasta into 13x9-inch baking dish. Stir gently; drizzle reserved cheese sauce over top. Cover and refrigerate 24 hours.

NEXT DAY, preheat oven to 350° F. Bake, covered for 1 hour and 10 minutes or until thoroughly heated and pasta is tender. Garnish with parsley, if desired. Serves 4.

Serve each with a 1-ounce breadstick.

Exchanges: 2½ meats, 2 breads, 2 vegetables, ½ milk, 2 fats

Flank Steak

1	lb. lean flank steak, trimmed of fat	1	tsp. bottled minced garlic
½	tsp. salt	1	tsp. olive oil
1	tsp. cracked or freshly ground pepper	2	tsp. balsamic vinegar
		1½	tbsp. fresh lemon juice

Rub steak with salt, pepper and garlic. Heat oil in large skillet over medium-high heat. Add steak; cook 6 minutes each side, or until desired doneness, basting with vinegar while cooking. Cut steak across grain into thin slices; drizzle lemon juice over pieces. Serves 4.

Serve each with 1 twice-baked potato and 1 cup steamed broccoli.

Exchanges: 3 meats, 2 breads, 1 vegetable, 1 fat

Philly Cheese Beef Sandwich

8	oz. cooked deli-style roast beef, thinly sliced	¼	tsp. black pepper
4	2-oz. hoagie-style rolls	4	1-oz. slices reduced-fat Swiss cheese
1	teaspoon olive oil		Olive-oil-flavored nonstick cooking spray
1½	c. sliced onion		
1½	c. sliced green bell pepper		

Preheat broiler. Heat oil in nonstick skillet over medium heat. Add onion; sauté 10 minutes, stirring frequently. Add bell pepper and black pepper; sauté 3 minutes more or until bell pepper is tender-crisp. Fill each roll with 2 ounces beef and 1/4 cup sautéed vegetables topped with 1 slice cheese. Place sandwiches on baking sheet coated with cooking spray; broil 2 minutes or until cheese melts.

Serve each with 1 cup **Broccoli Slaw**.

Exchanges: 3 meats, 2 breads, 1½ vegetables, 1 fat

Broccoli Slaw

1   16-oz. bag broccoli slaw mix, shredded
¼ c. sweet pickle relish
⅓ c. low-fat mayonnaise
1   tsp. prepared brown mustard
¼ tsp. celery seed
¼ tsp. black pepper

Combine all ingredients in large bowl; refrigerate until needed. Serves 4.

Exchanges: 3 meats, 2 breads, 1½ vegetables, 1 fat

~ ~

Grilled Tuna Steaks

4 4-oz. tuna steaks, about
    ½ in. thick
⅓ c. fresh lime juice
½ tsp. dried oregano
½ tsp. ground cumin
¼ tsp. salt

2 garlic cloves, minced
1 tsp. olive oil
1 tsp. cracked pepper
   Lime slices (optional)
   Nonstick cooking spray

Combine lime juice, oregano, cumin, salt and garlic in large shallow dish; mix well. Add tuna; turn to coat. Cover and marinate in refrigerator 1 hour, turning steaks occasionally.

Preheat broiler. Remove tuna from dish; discard marinade. Brush oil over steaks; sprinkle with pepper. Place fish on broiler pan coated with cooking spray; broil 5 minutes or until medium—do not turn. (Cook longer to desired doneness.) Garnish with lime slices, if desired.

Serve each with ½ cup roasted potatoes, 1 cup grilled vegetables and a 1-ounce dinner roll topped with 1 teaspoon reduced-fat margarine.

Exchanges: 3 meats, 2 breads, 2 vegetables, 1 fat

~ ~

Chicken with Garlic Gravy

1 2-lb. whole chicken	$\frac{1}{2}$ c. white cooking wine
1 tsp. dried thyme	1 10 $\frac{1}{2}$-oz. can low-salt
$\frac{1}{4}$ tsp. salt	chicken broth, divided
$\frac{1}{4}$ tsp. pepper	1 tbsp. all-purpose flour
10 garlic cloves, peeled	Nonstick cooking spray

Preheat oven to 325° F. Remove giblets and neck from chicken; discard. Rinse chicken under cold water; pat dry with paper towels. Trim excess fat. Starting at neck cavity, loosen skin from breast and drumsticks by inserting fingers, gently pushing between skin and meat. Rub thyme, salt and pepper on breasts and drumsticks under loosened skin; place 2 garlic cloves in body cavity. Lift wing tips up and over back; tuck under chicken. Set aside. Combine remaining garlic cloves, cooking wine and half of broth in shallow roasting pan lined with foil. Place chicken on cooking rack coated with cooking spray; place rack in foil-lined pan. Insert meat thermometer into meaty part of thigh, making sure not to touch bone. Bake 1 hour and 45 minutes or until thermometer registers 180° F. Discard skin; place chicken on a platter and set aside, reserving pan drippings. Keep chicken warm.

Place flour in small saucepan; gradually add remaining half of broth, stirring with whisk until blended; set aside. Place a small zip-top plastic bag inside 2-cup measuring cup. Pour pan drippings into bag; let stand 10 minutes (fat will rise to the top). Seal bag; carefully snip off bottom corner of bag. Drain drippings into broth mixture in saucepan, stopping before fat layer reaches opening; discard fat. Bring mixture to a boil; cook 1 minute or until thick, stirring constantly with a whisk. Arrange 3 ounces chicken topped with 3 tablespoons gravy for each serving. Serves 4.

Serve each with $\frac{2}{3}$ cup mashed potatoes, 1 cup cooked green beans and a 1-ounce dinner roll.

Exchanges: 3 meats, 2 breads, 2 vegetables, $\frac{1}{2}$ fat

Creole Chicken and Rice

4   4-oz. boneless, skinless
    chicken breasts
2   tsp. vegetable oil
⅔   c. low-salt chicken broth
¼   tsp. salt
⅛   tsp. crushed red pepper
1   14½-oz. can Cajun-style
    stewed tomatoes, undrained
    and chopped

2   garlic cloves, crushed
1   10-oz. pkg. frozen cut okra,
    thawed
1½ tbsp. all-purpose flour
2   tbsp. water
¼   tsp. hot sauce (e.g., Tabasco)
2   c. hot cooked long-grain rice

Heat oil in large nonstick skillet over medium-high heat. Add chicken; cook 2 minutes each side. Add broth, salt, pepper, tomatoes and garlic; cover, reduce heat and simmer 8 minutes or until chicken is done. Add okra; simmer, covered, 3 minutes more. In small bowl, combine flour and water, stirring with a whisk; add to skillet. Simmer, uncovered, 2 minutes or until thick. Stir in hot sauce. Serves 4.

Serve each with ¾ cup sauce and ½ cup rice.

Exchanges: 3 meats, 2 breads, 2 vegetables, ½ fat

~ ~

Chicken and Bowtie Pasta

4   4-oz. boneless, skinless
    chicken breasts
1   c. chicken broth
1   tbsp. water
½   tsp. cornstarch

½   6-oz. tub reduced-fat cream
    cheese with garlic and spices
3   c. hot cooked bowtie pasta
    Chopped fresh parsley

In large skillet, combine chicken and chicken broth. Bring to boil; cover, reduce heat and simmer 15 minutes, turning chicken after 8 minutes. Remove chicken from skillet; set aside and keep warm. Bring cooking liquid back to boil; cook 5 minutes or until reduced to ⅔ cup. In small bowl or cup, combine water and cornstarch; blend well and add to skillet. Bring to boil; cook 1 minute, stirring constantly. Add cream cheese; cook until well blended, stirring constantly with whisk. Serve each breast half over ¾ cup pasta; then top with ¾ cup sauce and garnish with parsley. Serves 4.

Serve each with 1 cup sautéed summer squash.

Exchanges: 3½ meats, 2½ breads, 2 vegetables, 1 fat

~ ~

Chicken and Pasta Primavera

1 lb. boneless, skinless chicken breast, cut into bite-size pieces
$\frac{2}{3}$ c. all-purpose flour
$\frac{1}{4}$ tsp. salt
$\frac{1}{4}$ tsp. pepper
$1\frac{1}{2}$ tbsp. olive oil
1 c. sliced mushrooms
2 c. broccoli florets
2 c. sliced yellow squash
$\frac{2}{3}$ c. diagonally-sliced carrots
4 garlic cloves, minced
$\frac{1}{4}$ c. chopped fresh basil
16 cherry tomatoes, halved
1 c. no-salt chicken broth
$\frac{2}{3}$ c. dry white wine
3 c. hot cooked linguine (about 3 oz. uncooked)
$\frac{1}{2}$ c. freshly grated Parmesan cheese
Nonstick cooking spray

Place flour in shallow dish. Dredge chicken in flour; sprinkle with salt and pepper. Heat oil in large nonstick skillet coated with cooking spray. Add chicken; stir-fry over medium heat 4 minutes or until browned. Add mushrooms, broccoli, squash, carrots and garlic; stir-fry 2 minutes more. Stir in basil and tomatoes; spoon mixture into a large bowl; set aside. Add broth and wine to skillet, scraping pan to loosen browned bits; bring to a boil. Combine broth, chicken and pasta; toss well and sprinkle with cheese. Serves 4.

Serve each with 1 cup green salad with 2 tablespoons low-fat dressing.
Exchanges: 3 meats, 2$\frac{1}{2}$ breads, 2 vegetables, 1 fat

CONVERSION CHART
EQUIVALENT IMPERIAL AND METRIC MEASUREMENTS

Liquid Measures

Fluid Ounces	U.S.	Imperial	Milliliters
	1 teaspoon	1 teaspoon	5
$\frac{1}{4}$	2 teaspoons	1 dessert spoon	7
$\frac{1}{2}$	1 tablespoon	1 tablespoon	15
1	2 tablespoons	2 tablespoons	28
2	$\frac{1}{4}$ cup	4 tablespoons	56
4	$\frac{1}{2}$ cup or $\frac{1}{4}$ pint		110
5		$\frac{1}{4}$ pint or 1 gill	140
6	$\frac{3}{4}$ cup		170
8	1 cup or $\frac{1}{2}$ pint		225
9			250 or $\frac{1}{4}$ liter
10	$1\frac{1}{4}$ cups	$\frac{1}{2}$ pint	280
12	$1\frac{1}{2}$ cups or $\frac{3}{4}$ pint		340
15		3/4 pint	420
16	2 cups or 1 pint		450
18	$2\frac{1}{4}$ cups		500 or $\frac{1}{2}$ liter
20	$2\frac{1}{2}$ cups	1 pint	560
24	3 cups or $1\frac{1}{2}$ pints		675
25		$1\frac{1}{4}$	700
30	$3\frac{3}{4}$ cups	$1\frac{1}{2}$ pints	840
32	4 cups		900
36	$4\frac{1}{2}$ cups		1000 or 1 liter
40	5 cups	2 pints or 1 quart	1120
48	6 cups or 3 pints		1350
50		$2\frac{1}{2}$ pints	1400

Solid Measures

U.S. and Imperial Measures		Metric Measures	
Ounces	Pounds	Grams	Kilos
1		28	
2		56	
3½		100	
4	¼	112	
5		140	
6		168	
8	½	225	
9		250	¼
12	¾	340	
16	1	450	
18		500	½
20	1¼	560	
24		675	
27		750	¾
32	2	900	
36	2¼	1000	1
40	2½	1100	
48	3	1350	
54		1500	1½
64	4	1800	
72	4½	2000	2
80	5	2250	2¼
100	6	2800	2¾

Oven Temperature Equivalents

Fahrenheit	Celsius	Gas Mark	Description
225	110	$\frac{1}{4}$	Cool
250	130	$\frac{1}{2}$	
275	140	1	Very Slow
300	150	2	
325	170	3	Slow
350	180	4	Moderate
375	190	5	
400	200	6	Moderately Hot
425	220	7	Fairly Hot
450	230	8	Hot
475	240	9	Very Hot
500	250	10	Extremely Hot

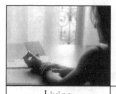

LEADER'S DISCUSSION GUIDE

Living
the Legacy

Week One: A Divine Inheritance

1. Invite group members to say Ephesians 1:4 in unison. Explain: Before the world even began, the Father knew about each one of you the great sacrifice His Son would make for you. Discuss: How does knowing this make you feel?

2. Briefly review the six gifts that Ephesians 1:1-14 describes as part of the Father's living will and testament: blessed, chosen, holy, predestined, adopted and forgiven. Discuss: Which of these most impacts you at this particular point in your spiritual pilgrimage?

3. **Before the meeting,** enlist a volunteer to tell how realizing that he or she has a precious inheritance from the heavenly Father is helping him or her deal with physical, emotional or spiritual issues. After this person shares, allow other group members an opportunity to share.

4. Explain: James 1:12 promises God will bless us if we persevere under trial. Invite members to tell how they believe God has blessed them during difficult times.

5. Form small groups of three or four. After reading Ephesians 1:4, assign the following question for group discussion: How does knowing that God expects you to live a holy and blameless life impact your decisions about how you take care of your body?

6. Instruct small groups to read Romans 8:28-30 and discuss (1) characteristics of a person whose heart is totally committed to Christ and (2) how members are seeking to conform to the likeness of Christ.

7. Reconvene the whole group. Allow a volunteer from each small group to summarize the discussion—avoiding any mention of personal information. Read this statement: Think about it! He knows the issues that spurred you to participate in First Place right now. Instruct members to close their eyes and silently reflect on this statement. Ask them to thank God for knowing and caring about them to such an extent.

8. Invite each person to pray a sentence prayer based on the gift he or she identified earlier in the session. An example would be: Thank You, God, for reminding me about how much You've forgiven me.

Week Two: Grace Still So Amazing

1. Select three volunteers to recite Ephesians 2:8-9 from memory.

2. Explain: God has the authority to leave us His matchless inheritance because of who He is. Invite volunteers to share their meditations on Colossians 1:15-17 and Hebrews 11:3,39 from Day 1.

3. Ask for responses to this statement: Grace is the utter generosity of God which He gives us as adopted children, even though as sinners we don't deserve it. Invite members to share testimonies of times when they have been especially aware of God's gift of grace in their lives.

4. Form small groups. Enlist a recorder from each group to take notes and prepare to report to the whole group. Instruct groups to discuss messages from the world that discourage a healthy lifestyle. Then have them contrast these messages with God's truths about caring for our bodies. After discussion, call for reports.

5. Explain: The role of good works in a person's faith is to honor God and to provide a testimony of the believer's living faith. Emphasize that our salvation is a free gift from God through Christ, not to be earned but to be accepted. Ask groups to (1) name good works that Christians try to use to cover painful memories or present weaknesses and (2) list ways to develop new habits that result in healthy lifestyles. Allow time for discussion.

6. Reconvene the whole group. Call for reports.

7. Discuss: In what practical ways would your life be different if you concentrated on God's work of grace in your life? On the board or newsprint, list responses (Examples: a forgiving spirit, expressing gratitude to God daily.) Explain: Making a conscious effort to be aware of God's grace each day will help these differences become reality.

8. Ask this question from the material in Day 5: Name the two qualities we possess through God's power (see Colossians 1:11-14). Then discuss: How are you relying on God to develop these qualities in your life? Allow time for several responses.

9. Invite several members to share ways the group encourages them to achieve their First Place goals. Then close in prayer thanking God for these encouragements. Remind members to pray for one another in the week ahead and to encourage another class member in some way.

Week Three: The Positive Power of Peace

1. Invite the group to recite Ephesians 2:14-15 in unison. Then instruct member to choose one of the memory verses from the previous two weeks and recite it to another group member. Discuss: How has an awareness of God's peace helped you keep your First Place commitments during the past week? Wait for responses.

2. Point out that Paul calls the dividing wall a "wall of hostility" (see Ephesians 2:14). Explain: We can often identify such walls in our lives by recognizing what makes us angry. As an example, share a wall that exists in your own life. Then invite volunteers to share dividing walls that exist in their lives. If, after several responses, health and fitness issues have not been mentioned, ask if these are (or have been) barriers between members and God. Stress group confidentiality.

3. As a group pray for the walls in one another's lives to be destroyed.

4. Discuss how Ephesians 2:15 relates to Matthew 5:17.

5. Read aloud the three passages from Day 3 (pp. 36-37) and relate them to God's peace. Invite members to identify the benefits of God's peace, especially as they relate to the First Place commitments.

6. Explain: God's peace gives you the ability to overcome any obstacles and to experience the benefits that have been mentioned. A person at peace is reconciled to God, to self and to others. Lead the group to characterize a person at peace. Record responses on the board.

7. Form small groups. Instruct them to discuss ways they can proclaim God's peace to persons who are (1) near and (2) far away. Then reconvene the whole group and present small-group reports.

8. If your group feels comfortable in sharing, ask how the memorization of Scriptures and using them in prayer have made a difference in their prayer life. If they have not yet begun to do so, challenge members to memorize one other verse of Scripture this next week and use it in their prayer time.

9. Close with a circle of prayer. Invite members to pray for the person on his or her right, asking God to help this person keep his or her commitments to a healthy lifestyle during the coming week.

Week Four: God's 100 Percent

1. Quote from memory Ephesians 3:19, then have volunteers quote it. Discuss: What difference would it make in your life to remember daily that you are filled to the measure of all the fullness of God?

2. Invite members to form pairs, or threesomes if necessary. Have them share ways their health or spiritual issues may have kept them from feeling Christ's love or the love of others. After the time of sharing, emphasize: *Nothing—not race, heritage or appearance —can separate us from Christ's love.* This is the truth of Romans 8:35-39.

3. Ask pairs to share changes they need to make in each of the areas listed.

4. Reconvene the whole group. Discuss: Do you now, or have you ever believed that living the Christian life involves depriving yourself of something you value? If so, what? Allow time for responses, then discuss: Why is following Christ not a deprivation? Summarize by explaining: Our only other choice—following Satan—leads to death and destruction (see John 10:10). Through Christ we experience a far better life.

5. Invite volunteers to share ways they experience a more abundant life because of Christ's presence in them. If anyone prayed to receive Christ as a result of this study, **prior to the meeting** ask that person to share the experience. Form a circle around the person and pray for guidance and blessings as he or she begins new life in Christ. Be sensitive to anyone in your group who is not a Christian.

6. Discuss: In Day 5 which of the nine commitments did you select to work on as a way to feel closer to God? Point out the futility of merely trying harder to please God. Read aloud Ephesians 3:16 and Philippians 4:12-13. Explain: These verses promise that God will give us the strength we need.

7. Instruct members to silently reflect on the question: What would it take for you to give God 100 percent regarding the proper care of your body? After a moment of silence, share a personal testimony about one way God is helping you reach your First Place goals.

8. Invite two volunteers to pray, asking God to supply the strength for group members to meet their First Place goals.

Week Five: Maturity—A Choice

1. **Before the meeting,** ask someone to prepare a brief testimony about his or her experience in putting off the old self and putting on the new self. As the session begins, ask a volunteer to quote the memory verse, Ephesians 4:22-24. Call on the previously enlisted member to share his or her testimony.

2. Discuss: Has there ever been a time when your foolishness as a Christian has been ridiculed by someone who does not know Christ? Allow time for responses; then continue: What are things you once considered foolishness that are now most precious to you?

3. Discuss the question posed in Day 2: In the care of your body, how do you sometimes live as one who does not know Christ? After a few responses, ask members to identify some traits of the old nature that we need to set aside and some traits of our new nature that we need to develop. On the board, list responses under the appropriate headings.

4. Form three small groups. Assign one of the following categories to each group; the natural person, the worldly Christian and the spiritual Christian. Have them discuss this question: What new insights about this type of person helped you understand yourself? Reconvene and allow time for small-group reports.

5. Discuss: What is the relationship between our minds and our actions? How does mastering our minds lead to healthy lifestyle habits? What does having the mind of Christ mean to you? (See 1 Corinthians 2:16.)

6. Invite members to share with one another the actions they identified that help them overcome the temptations that get them off track in reaching their goals in First Place.

7. Discuss: How do positive, optimistic thoughts encourage us to keep our commitments and reach our goals? Emphasize the role of Bible study and prayer in filling our minds with uplifting thoughts. Discuss how memorizing Scripture allows us to fill our minds with thoughts of Christ.

8. Discuss how the prayer journal can help members identify and reflect on answers to prayer. Invite other suggestions for filling our minds with Christ-honoring thoughts.

9. Lead the group in prayer. Thank God for the evidences of His work in members' lives. Mention specific examples that have been previously shared in the group.

Week Six: A Love Relationship

1. Bring wedding pictures of yourself or a family member for display in the room. Begin by asking volunteers to tell a humorous or meaningful event from a recent wedding they attended. Recall the story of Rachel in this week's introduction, and apply it to our love relationship with the Lord.

2. Invite volunteers to tell what the command to imitate God means to them (see Ephesians 5:1). After several responses, discuss: What is the relationship between our love for God and obedience to Him? Assign the following verses to be read aloud: Matthew 28:20, Luke 6:46, John 14:23-24 and 1 John 3:6,18.

3. Discuss: What is the relationship between love and forgiveness? Why does it grieve the Spirit when we are unforgiving? Have someone read Matthew 6:14-15. Point out that the most loving individuals are those who realize how much they have been forgiven (see Luke 7:47). If someone in the group is struggling with forgiveness, spend additional time in sharing and praying together. Allow those who have working through this issue to relate their experiences.

4. Invite members to share from Day 3 the specific ways they can show sacrificial love to others. Invite them to tell about ways others have befriended them. Discuss: What are some motives for befriending others that are self-serving? (To get attention, love, appreciation, etc.) Then ask: What distinguishes sacrificial from self-service love?

5. Make the transition to Day 4 by asking members to identify their favorite scent—whether perfume, food or flowers. Give them the opportunity to express how they feel about being sweet smelling to God. Lead the group to identify ways we smell sweet to God and ways we do not.

6. Invite volunteers to explain how they can live a more sacrificial lifestyle in order to achieve their First Place goals.

7. Discuss how memorizing Scriptures of praise helps them to praise God and be more aware of His greatness.

8. Conclude by offering a sacrifice of praise. Have members read the praises they wrote in response to Day 5. Close with prayers of praise.

Week Seven: Living in the Light

1. **Before the meeting,** assign three members one each of the three phrases in Ephesians 5:8 to explain to the group. As the session begins, repeat the verse as a group. Then call on the three enlisted members to explain the three phrases.

2. Explain: We who are in Christ have come out of the darkness into His light. Discuss: Why do you suppose some of us have difficulty seeing ourselves as children of light? (Possible answers include a negative self-concept, ongoing disobedience, or seeking to live in our own power.)

3. Form two groups. Ask one group to identify ways Christians reflect Christ's light. Ask the other group to identify ways Christians fail to reflect Christ's light. Reconvene the whole group and share reports.

4. Refer to Day 1 and discuss: Which characteristic—goodness, righteousness or truth—do you find most difficult to practice? What practical step did you identify to cultivate these fruits?

5. Discuss the following statement from Day 2: The only way to displace evil is to replace it. Solicit examples of replacing evil, such as choosing a family-oriented movie, apologizing to a friend, etc.

6. Ask for examples of the three ways to make the most of our time: live wisely, treat time as valuable and understand the Lord's will.

7. Discuss the following statement: What alcohol falsely promises, the Spirit delivers. Call on volunteers to share their descriptions of a person who is consistently being filled with the Spirit.

8. Discuss responses to the activity in which members were asked to list three reasons to be grateful and three things that challenge gratitude. Discuss: What character trait results from consistently choosing to practice gratitude? What are the results of focusing on our failures or those of others?

9. In closing, invite members to close their eyes and focus on Jesus as the source of all they have. Then ask each member to offer a brief sentence prayer of thanksgiving to God.

Week Eight: The Family of Faith

1. Repeat Ephesians 4:3. Discuss: How does last week's memory verse apply to the command to keep unity through peace?

2. Discuss this question from Day 1: Why are Christians often perceived as quarrelsome, arguing over anything from the color of carpet in the sanctuary to basic doctrines?

3. Discuss: Christians sometimes have difficulty dealing with the emotion of anger. Did anyone present grow up in a family in which angry displays were not permitted? If so, how did you learn to deal with your anger? Then invite anyone who grew up in a family in which anger was dealt with responsibly to share their experiences.

4. Review the four responses to anger discussed in the last learning activity in Day 2. Discuss: Which response most clearly describes your method of dealing with anger? Which response would you prefer to use in dealing with anger?

5. Have members make a list of reasons why they get angry. Discuss how we decide which issues should be confronted and which should be forgotten.

6. Read aloud Ephesians 5:29. Ask members which statement in Day 3 most nearly describes how they feel about their bodies. Then discuss: What could you do to better accept, nourish and care for your body? Affirm the fact that a member's participation in this group represents a meaningful effort to fulfill this goal.

7. Discuss: What character traits will children develop if they learn to disobey their parents? What character traits will they develop through disobedience? What character traits do we as Christian adults need to develop through obedience?

8. Review Ephesians 4:28 and 6:5-9. Discuss: What keywords or phrases did you identify that apply to your life and work situation? How can you more fully implement the truth of Ephesians 6:7 in your work life?

9. Lead members to pray for unity in the church, harmony in the family and an effective ministry through their work.

Week Nine: The Winning Side

1. Recite this week's memory verse. Remind members that the book of Ephesians is not just a feel-good epistle about God's goodness; it also contains a stern warning about Satan's attempts to keep us from remembering God's free gifts of inheritance. Invite members to share their feelings when they read the warning in Ephesians 6:12.

2. Explain: Today believers are often ridiculed for talking about Satan. Some do not even believe Satan is real. Share your convictions about this issue and allow time for members to voice opinions. Ask volunteers to share testimonies about times they believe Satan was at the root of a battle they faced. Discuss: How did you attempt to defeat the enemy in that situation?

3. Discuss the questions at the beginning of Day 2. After several responses, ask: What are some ways we can know that a person worships Satan? God? Discuss: How does knowing that God is more powerful than Satan help you resist temptation?

4. Read aloud 1 Peter 5:8-9. Invite volunteers to share practical examples of each command: be self-controlled, be alert, stand firm. Relate each of these commands to First Place commitments and goals.

5. Invite members to form pairs. Instruct each pair to discuss ways Satan seeks direct advantage over them by (1) an unforgiving attitude or (2) keeping them bound to past memories.

6. As pairs continue to share, ask them to identify actions they can take to achieve victory in Christ. Then direct them to conclude in prayer for each other.

7. Reconvene the whole group. Ask members to call out words that express how they feel when they realize Satan is a defeated enemy.

8. Lead the group in a closing prayer. Pray for boldness in confronting the enemy. Pray for Christ to be the only One we worship.

Week Ten: Keep On Praying

1. Recite this week's memory verse in unison. Instruct members to form pairs and share a favorite memory verse from this study. Express appreciation to those who have consistently memorized the verses and led out in repeating them during group discussions.

2. Discuss the purposes of prayer, relating them to the purposes of good communication in any relationship. Conclude by reminding members that prayer was God's idea and that both Jesus and Paul modeled a lifestyle of prayer. Explain: Although we may never understand how prayer brings about change, we know it does.

3. Discuss the meaning of "pray in the Spirit" (Ephesians 6:18). Then discuss the implications of praying "on all occasions," including times we may be discouraged, irritable or stressed. Encourage members to treat prayer as a discipline, not something to be attempted only when we feel like it.

4. Form four groups. Assign each group one letter from the ACTS acrostic. Ask groups to report back to the large group after discussing (1) what the letter stands for, (2) why this aspect of prayer is necessary, and (3) examples of prayers we can pray using this concept.

5. Instruct the small groups to spend some time in prayer. Suggest they say sentence prayers using each of the four elements of the ACTS acrostic.

6. Encourage members to share intercessory prayers that have been answered during the past 10 weeks. Encourage them to share other needs, which will be prayed for at the end of today's meeting.

7. Discuss the role of prayer in helping us to become bold witnesses. What is the basis for our boldness? What is the relationship between boldness and love? Read aloud 1 John 4:18.

8. Ask members to identify changes in their daily routines and lifestyles during the past 10 weeks. Discuss: How do you intend to continue living your legacy in Christ?

9. Discuss how Scripture memory has helped them in living for Christ. Invite members to share some of the methods they used to memorize verses. Ask volunteers to share other verses besides the ones they have memorized during this study.

10. Form a circle and pray for requests from members. Thank members for their participation. Close the meeting with appropriate words and expressions of appreciation and affection. Encourage members to use the verses they have memorized to tear down strongholds and build a stronger prayer life.

PERSONAL WEIGHT RECORD

Week	Weight	+ or -	Goal This Session	Pounds to Goal
1				
2				
3				
4				
5				
6				
7				
8				
9				
10				
11				
12				
13				
Final				

Beginning Measurements

Waist_____ Hips_____ Thighs_____ Chest_____

Ending Measurements

Waist_____ Hips_____ Thighs_____ Chest_____

COMMITMENT RECORDS

How to Fill Out a Commitment Record

The Commitment Record (CR) is an aid for you in keeping track of your accomplishments. Begin a new CR on the morning of the day your class meets. This ensures that your CR is complete before your next meeting. Turn in the CR weekly to your leader.

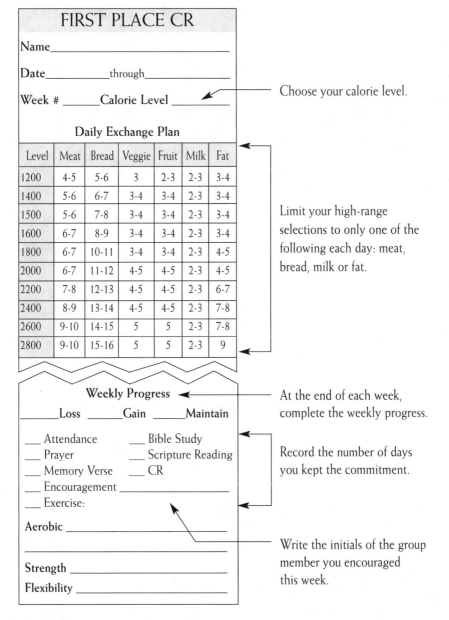

FIRST PLACE CR

Name_____

Date_____through_____

Week # _____Calorie Level _____

Choose your calorie level.

Daily Exchange Plan

Level	Meat	Bread	Veggie	Fruit	Milk	Fat
1200	4-5	5-6	3	2-3	2-3	3-4
1400	5-6	6-7	3-4	3-4	2-3	3-4
1500	5-6	7-8	3-4	3-4	2-3	3-4
1600	6-7	8-9	3-4	3-4	2-3	3-4
1800	6-7	10-11	3-4	3-4	2-3	4-5
2000	6-7	11-12	4-5	4-5	2-3	4-5
2200	7-8	12-13	4-5	4-5	2-3	6-7
2400	8-9	13-14	4-5	4-5	2-3	7-8
2600	9-10	14-15	5	5	2-3	7-8
2800	9-10	15-16	5	5	2-3	9

Limit your high-range selections to only one of the following each day: meat, bread, milk or fat.

Weekly Progress

_____Loss _____Gain _____Maintain

At the end of each week, complete the weekly progress.

___ Attendance   ___ Bible Study
___ Prayer   ___ Scripture Reading
___ Memory Verse   ___ CR
___ Encouragement _____
___ Exercise:

Aerobic _____

_____

Strength _____

Flexibility _____

Record the number of days you kept the commitment.

Write the initials of the group member you encouraged this week.

DAY 7: Date _____

Morning _____
_____
_____

Midday _____
_____
_____

Evening _____
_____
_____

Snacks _____
_____
_____

___ **Meat** _____   ☐ Prayer
___ **Bread** _____   ☐ Bible Study
___ **Vegetable** ____ ☐ Scripture Reading
___ **Fruit** _____   ☐ Memory Verse
___ **Milk** _____   ☐ Encouragement
___ **Fat** _____   ☐ Water_____

Exercise

Aerobic _____
_____

Strength _____

Flexibility _____

List the foods you have eaten. On this condensed CR it is not necessary to exchange each food choice. It will be the responsibility of each member that the tally marks you list below are accurate regarding each food choice. If you are unsure of an exchange, check the Live-It section of your copy of the *Member's Guide.*

List the daily food exchange choices to the left of the food groups.

Use tally marks for the actual food and water consumed.

Check off commitments completed. Use tally marks to record each 8-oz. serving of water.

List type and duration of exercise.

DAY 5: Date ___

Morning ___

Midday ___

Evening ___

Snacks ___

- Meat ___
- Bread ___
- Vegetable ___
- Fruit ___
- Milk ___
- Fat ___

☐ Prayer
☐ Bible Study
☐ Scripture Reading
☐ Memory Verse
☐ Encouragement

Water ___

Exercise
Aerobic ___

Strength ___
Flexibility ___

DAY 6: Date ___

Morning ___

Midday ___

Evening ___

Snacks ___

- Meat ___
- Bread ___
- Vegetable ___
- Fruit ___
- Milk ___
- Fat ___

☐ Prayer
☐ Bible Study
☐ Scripture Reading
☐ Memory Verse
☐ Encouragement

Water ___

Exercise
Aerobic ___

Strength ___
Flexibility ___

DAY 7: Date ___

Morning ___

Midday ___

Evening ___

Snacks ___

- Meat ___
- Bread ___
- Vegetable ___
- Fruit ___
- Milk ___
- Fat ___

☐ Prayer
☐ Bible Study
☐ Scripture Reading
☐ Memory Verse
☐ Encouragement

Water ___

Exercise
Aerobic ___

Strength ___
Flexibility ___

FIRST PLACE CR

Name ___
Date ___ through ___
Week # ___ Calorie Level ___

Daily Exchange Plan

Level	Meat	Bread	Veggie	Fruit	Milk	Fat
1200	4-5	5-6	3	2-3	2-3	3-4
1400	5-6	6-7	3-4	3-4	2-3	3-4
1500	5-6	7-8	3-4	3-4	2-3	3-4
1600	6-7	8-9	3-4	3-4	2-3	3-4
1800	6-7	10-11	3-4	3-4	2-3	4-5
2000	6-7	11-12	4-5	4-5	2-3	4-5
2200	7-8	12-13	4-5	4-5	2-3	6-7
2400	8-9	13-14	4-5	4-5	2-3	7-8
2600	9-10	14-15	5	5	2-3	7-8
2800	9-10	15-16	5	5	2-3	9

You may always choose the high range of vegetables and fruits. Limit your high range selections to only one of the following: meat, bread, milk or fat.

Weekly Progress

___ Loss ___ Gain ___ Maintain

___ Attendance ___ Bible Study
___ Prayer ___ Scripture Reading
___ Memory Verse ___ CR
___ Encouragement:
___ Exercise
Aerobic ___

Strength ___
Flexibility ___

DAY 1: Date _____

Morning _____

Midday _____

Evening _____

Snacks _____

___ Meat	☐ Prayer
___ Bread	☐ Bible Study
___ Vegetable	☐ Scripture Reading
___ Fruit	☐ Memory Verse
___ Milk	☐ Encouragement
___ Fat	___ Water

Exercise
Aerobic _____

Strength _____

Flexibility _____

DAY 2: Date _____

Morning _____

Midday _____

Evening _____

Snacks _____

___ Meat	☐ Prayer
___ Bread	☐ Bible Study
___ Vegetable	☐ Scripture Reading
___ Fruit	☐ Memory Verse
___ Milk	☐ Encouragement
___ Fat	___ Water

Exercise
Aerobic _____

Strength _____

Flexibility _____

DAY 3: Date _____

Morning _____

Midday _____

Evening _____

Snacks _____

___ Meat	☐ Prayer
___ Bread	☐ Bible Study
___ Vegetable	☐ Scripture Reading
___ Fruit	☐ Memory Verse
___ Milk	☐ Encouragement
___ Fat	___ Water

Exercise
Aerobic _____

Strength _____

Flexibility _____

DAY 4: Date _____

Morning _____

Midday _____

Evening _____

Snacks _____

___ Meat	☐ Prayer
___ Bread	☐ Bible Study
___ Vegetable	☐ Scripture Reading
___ Fruit	☐ Memory Verse
___ Milk	☐ Encouragement
___ Fat	___ Water

Exercise
Aerobic _____

Strength _____

Flexibility _____

FIRST PLACE CR

Name _____

Date _____ through _____

Week # _____ Calorie Level _____

Daily Exchange Plan

Level	Meat	Bread	Veggie	Fruit	Milk	Fat
1200	4-5	5-6	3	2-3	2-3	3-4
1400	5-6	6-7	3-4	3-4	2-3	3-4
1500	5-6	7-8	3-4	3-4	2-3	3-4
1600	6-7	8-9	3-4	3-4	2-3	3-4
1800	6-7	10-11	3-4	3-4	2-3	4-5
2000	6-7	11-12	4-5	4-5	2-3	4-5
2200	7-8	12-13	4-5	4-5	2-3	6-7
2400	8-9	13-14	4-5	4-5	2-3	7-8
2600	9-10	14-15	5	5	2-3	7-8
2800	9-10	15-16	5	5	2-3	9

You may always choose the high range of vegetables and fruits. Limit your high range selections to only one of the following: meat, bread, milk or fat.

_____ Loss _____ Gain _____ Maintain

_____ Attendance _____ Bible Study
_____ Prayer _____ Scripture Reading
_____ Memory Verse _____ CR
_____ Encouragement
_____ Exercise
Aerobic _____

Strength _____
Flexibility _____

DAY 5: Date _____

Morning _____

Midday _____

Evening _____

Snacks _____

_____ Meat ☐ Prayer
_____ Bread ☐ Bible Study
_____ Vegetable ☐ Scripture Reading
_____ Fruit ☐ Memory Verse
_____ Milk ☐ Encouragement
_____ Fat _____ Water
Exercise
Aerobic _____

Strength _____
Flexibility _____

DAY 6: Date _____

Morning _____

Midday _____

Evening _____

Snacks _____

_____ Meat ☐ Prayer
_____ Bread ☐ Bible Study
_____ Vegetable ☐ Scripture Reading
_____ Fruit ☐ Memory Verse
_____ Milk ☐ Encouragement
_____ Fat _____ Water
Exercise
Aerobic _____

Strength _____
Flexibility _____

DAY 7: Date _____

Morning _____

Midday _____

Evening _____

Snacks _____

_____ Meat ☐ Prayer
_____ Bread ☐ Bible Study
_____ Vegetable ☐ Scripture Reading
_____ Fruit ☐ Memory Verse
_____ Milk ☐ Encouragement
_____ Fat _____ Water
Exercise
Aerobic _____

Strength _____
Flexibility _____

DAY 1: Date _____

Morning _____

Midday _____

Evening _____

Snacks _____

___ Meat	☐ Prayer
___ Bread	☐ Bible Study
___ Vegetable	☐ Scripture Reading
___ Fruit	☐ Memory Verse
___ Milk	☐ Encouragement
___ Fat	___ Water

Exercise
Aerobic _____
Strength _____
Flexibility _____

DAY 2: Date _____

Morning _____

Midday _____

Evening _____

Snacks _____

___ Meat	☐ Prayer
___ Bread	☐ Bible Study
___ Vegetable	☐ Scripture Reading
___ Fruit	☐ Memory Verse
___ Milk	☐ Encouragement
___ Fat	___ Water

Exercise
Aerobic _____
Strength _____
Flexibility _____

DAY 3: Date _____

Morning _____

Midday _____

Evening _____

Snacks _____

___ Meat	☐ Prayer
___ Bread	☐ Bible Study
___ Vegetable	☐ Scripture Reading
___ Fruit	☐ Memory Verse
___ Milk	☐ Encouragement
___ Fat	___ Water

Exercise
Aerobic _____
Strength _____
Flexibility _____

DAY 4: Date _____

Morning _____

Midday _____

Evening _____

Snacks _____

___ Meat	☐ Prayer
___ Bread	☐ Bible Study
___ Vegetable	☐ Scripture Reading
___ Fruit	☐ Memory Verse
___ Milk	☐ Encouragement
___ Fat	___ Water

Exercise
Aerobic _____
Strength _____
Flexibility _____

FIRST PLACE CR

Name _____

Date _____ through _____

Week # _____ Calorie Level _____

Daily Exchange Plan

Level	Meat	Bread	Veggie	Fruit	Milk	Fat
1200	4-5	5-6	3	2-3	2-3	3-4
1400	5-6	6-7	3-4	3-4	2-3	3-4
1500	5-6	7-8	3-4	3-4	2-3	3-4
1600	6-7	8-9	3-4	3-4	2-3	3-4
1800	6-7	10-11	3-4	3-4	2-3	4-5
2000	6-7	11-12	4-5	4-5	2-3	4-5
2200	7-8	12-13	4-5	4-5	2-3	6-7
2400	8-9	13-14	4-5	4-5	2-3	7-8
2600	9-10	14-15	5	5	2-3	7-8
2800	9-10	15-16	5	5	2-3	9

You may always choose the high range of vegetables and fruits. Limit your high range selections to only one of the following: meat, bread, milk or fat.

_____ Loss _____ Gain _____ Maintain

_____ Attendance _____ Bible Study
_____ Prayer _____ Scripture Reading
_____ Memory Verse _____ CR
_____ Encouragement
_____ Exercise
Aerobic _____

Strength _____
Flexibility _____

DAY 5: Date _____

Morning _____

Midday _____

Evening _____

Snacks _____

_____ Meat   ☐ Prayer
_____ Bread   ☐ Bible Study
_____ Vegetable ☐ Scripture Reading
_____ Fruit   ☐ Memory Verse
_____ Milk   ☐ Encouragement
_____ Fat   Water _____

Exercise
Aerobic _____

Strength _____
Flexibility _____

DAY 6: Date _____

Morning _____

Midday _____

Evening _____

Snacks _____

_____ Meat   ☐ Prayer
_____ Bread   ☐ Bible Study
_____ Vegetable ☐ Scripture Reading
_____ Fruit   ☐ Memory Verse
_____ Milk   ☐ Encouragement
_____ Fat   Water _____

Exercise
Aerobic _____

Strength _____
Flexibility _____

DAY 7: Date _____

Morning _____

Midday _____

Evening _____

Snacks _____

_____ Meat   ☐ Prayer
_____ Bread   ☐ Bible Study
_____ Vegetable ☐ Scripture Reading
_____ Fruit   ☐ Memory Verse
_____ Milk   ☐ Encouragement
_____ Fat   Water _____

Exercise
Aerobic _____

Strength _____
Flexibility _____

DAY 1: Date _____

Morning _____

_____

Midday _____

_____

Evening _____

_____

Snacks _____

_____

_____

☐ Prayer		
____ Meat	____ Bread	☐ Bible Study
____ Vegetable		☐ Scripture Reading
____ Fruit		☐ Memory Verse
____ Milk		☐ Encouragement
____ Fat	____ Water	

Exercise
Aerobic _____
Strength _____
Flexibility _____

DAY 2: Date _____

Morning _____

_____

Midday _____

_____

Evening _____

_____

Snacks _____

_____

_____

☐ Prayer		
____ Meat	____ Bread	☐ Bible Study
____ Vegetable		☐ Scripture Reading
____ Fruit		☐ Memory Verse
____ Milk		☐ Encouragement
____ Fat	____ Water	

Exercise
Aerobic _____
Strength _____
Flexibility _____

DAY 3: Date _____

Morning _____

_____

Midday _____

_____

Evening _____

_____

Snacks _____

_____

_____

☐ Prayer		
____ Meat	____ Bread	☐ Bible Study
____ Vegetable		☐ Scripture Reading
____ Fruit		☐ Memory Verse
____ Milk		☐ Encouragement
____ Fat	____ Water	

Exercise
Aerobic _____
Strength _____
Flexibility _____

DAY 4: Date _____

Morning _____

_____

Midday _____

_____

Evening _____

_____

Snacks _____

_____

_____

☐ Prayer		
____ Meat	____ Bread	☐ Bible Study
____ Vegetable		☐ Scripture Reading
____ Fruit		☐ Memory Verse
____ Milk		☐ Encouragement
____ Fat	____ Water	

Exercise
Aerobic _____
Strength _____
Flexibility _____

FIRST PLACE CR

Name _____

Date _____ through _____

Week # _____ Calorie Level _____

Daily Exchange Plan

Level	Meat	Bread	Veggie	Fruit	Milk	Fat
1200	4-5	5-6	3	2-3	2-3	3-4
1400	5-6	6-7	3-4	3-4	2-3	3-4
1500	5-6	7-8	3-4	3-4	2-3	3-4
1600	6-7	8-9	3-4	3-4	2-3	3-4
1800	6-7	10-11	3-4	3-4	2-3	4-5
2000	6-7	11-12	4-5	4-5	2-3	4-5
2200	7-8	12-13	4-5	4-5	2-3	6-7
2400	8-9	13-14	4-5	4-5	2-3	7-8
2600	9-10	14-15	5	5	2-3	7-8
2800	9-10	15-16	5	5	2-3	9

You may always choose the high range of vegetables and fruits. Limit your high range selections to only one of the following: meat, bread, milk or fat.

_____ Loss _____ Gain _____ Maintain

_____ Attendance _____ Bible Study
_____ Prayer _____ Scripture Reading
_____ Memory Verse _____ CR
_____ Encouragement
_____ Exercise
_____ Aerobic

_____ Strength
_____ Flexibility

DAY 5: Date _____

Morning _____

Midday _____

Evening _____

Snacks _____

_____ Meat _____ ☐ Prayer
_____ Bread _____ ☐ Bible Study
_____ Vegetable _____ ☐ Scripture Reading
_____ Fruit _____ ☐ Memory Verse
_____ Milk _____ ☐ Encouragement
_____ Fat _____ Water _____

Exercise
Aerobic _____

Strength _____
Flexibility _____

DAY 6: Date _____

Morning _____

Midday _____

Evening _____

Snacks _____

_____ Meat _____ ☐ Prayer
_____ Bread _____ ☐ Bible Study
_____ Vegetable _____ ☐ Scripture Reading
_____ Fruit _____ ☐ Memory Verse
_____ Milk _____ ☐ Encouragement
_____ Fat _____ Water _____

Exercise
Aerobic _____

Strength _____
Flexibility _____

DAY 7: Date _____

Morning _____

Midday _____

Evening _____

Snacks _____

_____ Meat _____ ☐ Prayer
_____ Bread _____ ☐ Bible Study
_____ Vegetable _____ ☐ Scripture Reading
_____ Fruit _____ ☐ Memory Verse
_____ Milk _____ ☐ Encouragement
_____ Fat _____ Water _____

Exercise
Aerobic _____

Strength _____
Flexibility _____

DAY 1: Date _____

Morning _____

Midday _____

Evening _____

Snacks _____

___ Meat	☐ Prayer
___ Bread	☐ Bible Study
___ Vegetable	☐ Scripture Reading
___ Fruit	☐ Memory Verse
___ Milk	☐ Encouragement
___ Fat	___ Water

Exercise
Aerobic _____
Strength _____
Flexibility _____

DAY 2: Date _____

Morning _____

Midday _____

Evening _____

Snacks _____

___ Meat	☐ Prayer
___ Bread	☐ Bible Study
___ Vegetable	☐ Scripture Reading
___ Fruit	☐ Memory Verse
___ Milk	☐ Encouragement
___ Fat	___ Water

Exercise
Aerobic _____
Strength _____
Flexibility _____

DAY 3: Date _____

Morning _____

Midday _____

Evening _____

Snacks _____

___ Meat	☐ Prayer
___ Bread	☐ Bible Study
___ Vegetable	☐ Scripture Reading
___ Fruit	☐ Memory Verse
___ Milk	☐ Encouragement
___ Fat	___ Water

Exercise
Aerobic _____
Strength _____
Flexibility _____

DAY 4: Date _____

Morning _____

Midday _____

Evening _____

Snacks _____

___ Meat	☐ Prayer
___ Bread	☐ Bible Study
___ Vegetable	☐ Scripture Reading
___ Fruit	☐ Memory Verse
___ Milk	☐ Encouragement
___ Fat	___ Water

Exercise
Aerobic _____
Strength _____
Flexibility _____

FIRST PLACE CR

Name _____

Date _____ through _____

Date _____ Calorie Level _____

Week # _____

Daily Exchange Plan

Level	Meat	Bread	Veggie	Fruit	Milk	Fat
1200	4-5	5-6	3	2-3	2-3	3-4
1400	5-6	6-7	3-4	3-4	2-3	3-4
1500	5-6	7-8	3-4	3-4	2-3	3-4
1600	6-7	8-9	3-4	3-4	2-3	3-4
1800	6-7	10-11	3-4	3-4	2-3	4-5
2000	6-7	11-12	4-5	4-5	2-3	4-5
2200	7-8	12-13	4-5	4-5	2-3	6-7
2400	8-9	13-14	4-5	4-5	2-3	7-8
2600	9-10	14-15	5	5	2-3	7-8
2800	9-10	15-16	5	5	2-3	9

You may always choose the high range of vegetables and fruits. Limit your high range selections to only one of the following: meat, bread, milk or fat.

_____ Loss _____ Gain _____ Maintain

_____ Attendance _____ Bible Study
_____ Prayer _____ Scripture Reading
_____ Memory Verse _____ CR
_____ Encouragement
_____ Exercise
_____ Aerobic

_____ Strength
_____ Flexibility

DAY 5: Date _____

Morning _____

Midday _____

Evening _____

Snacks _____

_____ Meat ☐ Prayer
_____ Bread ☐ Bible Study
_____ Vegetable ☐ Scripture Reading
_____ Fruit ☐ Memory Verse
_____ Milk ☐ Encouragement
_____ Fat Water _____

Exercise
Aerobic _____

Strength _____
Flexibility _____

DAY 6: Date _____

Morning _____

Midday _____

Evening _____

Snacks _____

_____ Meat ☐ Prayer
_____ Bread ☐ Bible Study
_____ Vegetable ☐ Scripture Reading
_____ Fruit ☐ Memory Verse
_____ Milk ☐ Encouragement
_____ Fat Water _____

Exercise
Aerobic _____

Strength _____
Flexibility _____

DAY 7: Date _____

Morning _____

Midday _____

Evening _____

Snacks _____

_____ Meat ☐ Prayer
_____ Bread ☐ Bible Study
_____ Vegetable ☐ Scripture Reading
_____ Fruit ☐ Memory Verse
_____ Milk ☐ Encouragement
_____ Fat Water _____

Exercise
Aerobic _____

Strength _____
Flexibility _____

DAY 1: Date _____

Morning _____

Midday _____

Evening _____

Snacks _____

____ Meat	☐ Prayer
____ Bread	☐ Bible Study
____ Vegetable	☐ Scripture Reading
____ Fruit	☐ Memory Verse
____ Milk	☐ Encouragement
____ Fat	____ Water

Exercise
Aerobic _____
Strength _____
Flexibility _____

DAY 2: Date _____

Morning _____

Midday _____

Evening _____

Snacks _____

____ Meat	☐ Prayer
____ Bread	☐ Bible Study
____ Vegetable	☐ Scripture Reading
____ Fruit	☐ Memory Verse
____ Milk	☐ Encouragement
____ Fat	____ Water

Exercise
Aerobic _____
Strength _____
Flexibility _____

DAY 3: Date _____

Morning _____

Midday _____

Evening _____

Snacks _____

____ Meat	☐ Prayer
____ Bread	☐ Bible Study
____ Vegetable	☐ Scripture Reading
____ Fruit	☐ Memory Verse
____ Milk	☐ Encouragement
____ Fat	____ Water

Exercise
Aerobic _____
Strength _____
Flexibility _____

DAY 4: Date _____

Morning _____

Midday _____

Evening _____

Snacks _____

____ Meat	☐ Prayer
____ Bread	☐ Bible Study
____ Vegetable	☐ Scripture Reading
____ Fruit	☐ Memory Verse
____ Milk	☐ Encouragement
____ Fat	____ Water

Exercise
Aerobic _____
Strength _____
Flexibility _____

Name _____

Date _____ through _____

Week # _____ Calorie Level _____

Daily Exchange Plan

Level	Meat	Bread	Veggie	Fruit	Milk	Fat
1200	4-5	5-6	3	2-3	2-3	3-4
1400	5-6	6-7	3-4	3-4	2-3	3-4
1500	5-6	7-8	3-4	3-4	2-3	3-4
1600	6-7	8-9	3-4	3-4	2-3	3-4
1800	6-7	10-11	3-4	3-4	2-3	4-5
2000	6-7	11-12	4-5	4-5	2-3	4-5
2200	7-8	12-13	4-5	4-5	2-3	6-7
2400	8-9	13-14	4-5	4-5	2-3	7-8
2600	9-10	14-15	5	5	2-3	7-8
2800	9-10	15-16	5	5	2-3	9

You may always choose the high range of vegetables and fruits. Limit your high range selections to only one of the following: meat, bread, milk or fat.

_____ Loss _____ Gain _____ Maintain

_____ Attendance _____ Bible Study
_____ Prayer _____ Scripture Reading
_____ Memory Verse _____ CR
_____ Encouragement
_____ Exercise
_____ Aerobic

_____ Strength
_____ Flexibility

DAY 5: Date _____

Morning _____

Midday _____

Evening _____

Snacks _____

_____ Meat
_____ Bread
_____ Vegetable
_____ Fruit
_____ Milk
_____ Fat

☐ Prayer
☐ Bible Study
☐ Scripture Reading
☐ Memory Verse
☐ Encouragement
_____ Water

Exercise
Aerobic _____

Strength _____
Flexibility _____

DAY 6: Date _____

Morning _____

Midday _____

Evening _____

Snacks _____

_____ Meat
_____ Bread
_____ Vegetable
_____ Fruit
_____ Milk
_____ Fat

☐ Prayer
☐ Bible Study
☐ Scripture Reading
☐ Memory Verse
☐ Encouragement
_____ Water

Exercise
Aerobic _____

Strength _____
Flexibility _____

DAY 7: Date _____

Morning _____

Midday _____

Evening _____

Snacks _____

_____ Meat
_____ Bread
_____ Vegetable
_____ Fruit
_____ Milk
_____ Fat

☐ Prayer
☐ Bible Study
☐ Scripture Reading
☐ Memory Verse
☐ Encouragement
_____ Water

Exercise
Aerobic _____

Strength _____
Flexibility _____

DAY 1: Date _____

Morning _____

Midday _____

Evening _____

Snacks _____

- ☐ Prayer
- ☐ Bible Study
- ☐ Scripture Reading
- ☐ Memory Verse
- ☐ Encouragement

_____ Meat
_____ Bread
_____ Vegetable
_____ Fruit
_____ Milk
_____ Fat
_____ Water

Exercise
Aerobic _____
Strength _____
Flexibility _____

DAY 2: Date _____

Morning _____

Midday _____

Evening _____

Snacks _____

- ☐ Prayer
- ☐ Bible Study
- ☐ Scripture Reading
- ☐ Memory Verse
- ☐ Encouragement

_____ Meat
_____ Bread
_____ Vegetable
_____ Fruit
_____ Milk
_____ Fat
_____ Water

Exercise
Aerobic _____
Strength _____
Flexibility _____

DAY 3: Date _____

Morning _____

Midday _____

Evening _____

Snacks _____

- ☐ Prayer
- ☐ Bible Study
- ☐ Scripture Reading
- ☐ Memory Verse
- ☐ Encouragement

_____ Meat
_____ Bread
_____ Vegetable
_____ Fruit
_____ Milk
_____ Fat
_____ Water

Exercise
Aerobic _____
Strength _____
Flexibility _____

DAY 4: Date _____

Morning _____

Midday _____

Evening _____

Snacks _____

- ☐ Prayer
- ☐ Bible Study
- ☐ Scripture Reading
- ☐ Memory Verse
- ☐ Encouragement

_____ Meat
_____ Bread
_____ Vegetable
_____ Fruit
_____ Milk
_____ Fat
_____ Water

Exercise
Aerobic _____
Strength _____
Flexibility _____

Name _____

Date _____ through_____

Week # _____ Calorie Level _____

Daily Exchange Plan

Level	Meat	Bread	Veggie	Fruit	Milk	Fat
1200	4-5	5-6	3	2-3	2-3	3-4
1400	5-6	6-7	3-4	3-4	2-3	3-4
1500	5-6	7-8	3-4	3-4	2-3	3-4
1600	6-7	8-9	3-4	3-4	2-3	3-4
1800	6-7	10-11	3-4	3-4	2-3	4-5
2000	6-7	11-12	4-5	4-5	2-3	4-5
2200	7-8	12-13	4-5	4-5	2-3	6-7
2400	8-9	13-14	4-5	4-5	2-3	7-8
2600	9-10	14-15	5	5	2-3	7-8
2800	9-10	15-16	5	5	2-3	9

You may always choose the high range of vegetables and fruits. Limit your high range selections to only one of the following: meat, bread, milk or fat.

_____ Loss _____ Gain _____ Maintain

_____ Attendance _____ Bible Study
_____ Prayer _____ Scripture Reading
_____ Memory Verse _____ CR
_____ Encouragement
_____ Exercise
Aerobic

Strength _____
Flexibility _____

DAY 7: Date _____

Morning _____
_____

Midday _____
_____

Evening _____
_____

Snacks _____
_____

_____ Meat ☐ Prayer
_____ Bread ☐ Bible Study
_____ Vegetable ☐ Scripture Reading
_____ Fruit ☐ Memory Verse
_____ Milk ☐ Encouragement
_____ Fat ☐ Water _____

Exercise
Aerobic _____

Strength _____
Flexibility _____

DAY 6: Date _____

Morning _____
_____

Midday _____
_____

Evening _____
_____

Snacks _____
_____

_____ Meat ☐ Prayer
_____ Bread ☐ Bible Study
_____ Vegetable ☐ Scripture Reading
_____ Fruit ☐ Memory Verse
_____ Milk ☐ Encouragement
_____ Fat ☐ Water _____

Exercise
Aerobic _____

Strength _____
Flexibility _____

DAY 5: Date _____

Morning _____
_____

Midday _____
_____

Evening _____
_____

Snacks _____
_____

_____ Meat ☐ Prayer
_____ Bread ☐ Bible Study
_____ Vegetable ☐ Scripture Reading
_____ Fruit ☐ Memory Verse
_____ Milk ☐ Encouragement
_____ Fat ☐ Water _____

Exercise
Aerobic _____

Strength _____
Flexibility _____

DAY 1: Date _____

Morning _____

Midday _____

Evening _____

Snacks _____

___ Meat	☐ Prayer
___ Bread	☐ Bible Study
___ Vegetable	☐ Scripture Reading
___ Fruit	☐ Memory Verse
___ Milk	☐ Encouragement
___ Fat	___ Water

Exercise
Aerobic _____
Strength _____
Flexibility _____

DAY 2: Date _____

Morning _____

Midday _____

Evening _____

Snacks _____

___ Meat	☐ Prayer
___ Bread	☐ Bible Study
___ Vegetable	☐ Scripture Reading
___ Fruit	☐ Memory Verse
___ Milk	☐ Encouragement
___ Fat	___ Water

Exercise
Aerobic _____
Strength _____
Flexibility _____

DAY 3: Date _____

Morning _____

Midday _____

Evening _____

Snacks _____

___ Meat	☐ Prayer
___ Bread	☐ Bible Study
___ Vegetable	☐ Scripture Reading
___ Fruit	☐ Memory Verse
___ Milk	☐ Encouragement
___ Fat	___ Water

Exercise
Aerobic _____
Strength _____
Flexibility _____

DAY 4: Date _____

Morning _____

Midday _____

Evening _____

Snacks _____

___ Meat	☐ Prayer
___ Bread	☐ Bible Study
___ Vegetable	☐ Scripture Reading
___ Fruit	☐ Memory Verse
___ Milk	☐ Encouragement
___ Fat	___ Water

Exercise
Aerobic _____
Strength _____
Flexibility _____

FIRST PLACE CR

Daily Exchange Plan

Level	Meat	Bread	Veggie	Fruit	Milk	Fat
1200	4-5	5-6	3	2-3	2-3	3-4
1400	5-6	6-7	3-4	3-4	2-3	3-4
1500	5-6	7-8	3-4	3-4	2-3	3-4
1600	6-7	8-9	3-4	3-4	2-3	3-4
1800	6-7	10-11	3-4	3-4	2-3	4-5
2000	6-7	11-12	4-5	4-5	2-3	4-5
2200	7-8	12-13	4-5	4-5	2-3	6-7
2400	8-9	13-14	4-5	4-5	2-3	7-8
2600	9-10	14-15	5	5	2-3	7-8
2800	9-10	15-16	5	5	2-3	9

You may always choose the high range of vegetables and fruits. Limit your high range selections to only one of the following: meat, bread, milk or fat.

_____ Loss _____ Gain _____ Maintain

_____ Attendance _____ Bible Study
_____ Prayer _____ Scripture Reading
_____ Memory Verse _____ CR
_____ Encouragement
_____ Exercise
_____ Aerobic

_____ Strength
_____ Flexibility

DAY 5: Date _____

Morning _____

Midday _____

Evening _____

Snacks _____

_____ Meat   ☐ Prayer
_____ Bread   ☐ Bible Study
_____ Vegetable   ☐ Scripture Reading
_____ Fruit   ☐ Memory Verse
_____ Milk   ☐ Encouragement
_____ Fat   _____ Water

Exercise
Aerobic _____

Strength _____
Flexibility _____

DAY 6: Date _____

Morning _____

Midday _____

Evening _____

Snacks _____

_____ Meat   ☐ Prayer
_____ Bread   ☐ Bible Study
_____ Vegetable   ☐ Scripture Reading
_____ Fruit   ☐ Memory Verse
_____ Milk   ☐ Encouragement
_____ Fat   _____ Water

Exercise
Aerobic _____

Strength _____
Flexibility _____

DAY 7: Date _____

Morning _____

Midday _____

Evening _____

Snacks _____

_____ Meat   ☐ Prayer
_____ Bread   ☐ Bible Study
_____ Vegetable   ☐ Scripture Reading
_____ Fruit   ☐ Memory Verse
_____ Milk   ☐ Encouragement
_____ Fat   _____ Water

Exercise
Aerobic _____

Strength _____
Flexibility _____

DAY 1: Date _____

Morning _____

Midday _____

Evening _____

Snacks _____

___ Meat	☐ Prayer
___ Bread	☐ Bible Study
___ Vegetable	☐ Scripture Reading
___ Fruit	☐ Memory Verse
___ Milk	☐ Encouragement
___ Fat ___ Water	

Exercise
Aerobic _____
Strength _____
Flexibility _____

DAY 2: Date _____

Morning _____

Midday _____

Evening _____

Snacks _____

___ Meat	☐ Prayer
___ Bread	☐ Bible Study
___ Vegetable	☐ Scripture Reading
___ Fruit	☐ Memory Verse
___ Milk	☐ Encouragement
___ Fat ___ Water	

Exercise
Aerobic _____
Strength _____
Flexibility _____

DAY 3: Date _____

Morning _____

Midday _____

Evening _____

Snacks _____

___ Meat	☐ Prayer
___ Bread	☐ Bible Study
___ Vegetable	☐ Scripture Reading
___ Fruit	☐ Memory Verse
___ Milk	☐ Encouragement
___ Fat ___ Water	

Exercise
Aerobic _____
Strength _____
Flexibility _____

DAY 4: Date _____

Morning _____

Midday _____

Evening _____

Snacks _____

___ Meat	☐ Prayer
___ Bread	☐ Bible Study
___ Vegetable	☐ Scripture Reading
___ Fruit	☐ Memory Verse
___ Milk	☐ Encouragement
___ Fat ___ Water	

Exercise
Aerobic _____
Strength _____
Flexibility _____

Name _____

Date _____ through _____

Week # _____ Calorie Level _____

Daily Exchange Plan

Level	Meat	Bread	Veggie	Fruit	Milk	Fat
1200	4-5	5-6	3	2-3	2-3	3-4
1400	5-6	6-7	3-4	3-4	2-3	3-4
1500	5-6	7-8	3-4	3-4	2-3	3-4
1600	6-7	8-9	3-4	3-4	2-3	3-4
1800	6-7	10-11	3-4	3-4	2-3	4-5
2000	6-7	11-12	4-5	4-5	2-3	4-5
2200	7-8	12-13	4-5	4-5	2-3	6-7
2400	8-9	13-14	4-5	4-5	2-3	7-8
2600	9-10	14-15	5	5	2-3	7-8
2800	9-10	15-16	5	5	2-3	9

You may always choose the high range of vegetables and fruits. Limit your high range selections to only one of the following: meat, bread, milk or fat.

_____ Loss _____ Gain _____ Maintain
_____ Attendance _____ Bible Study
_____ Prayer _____ Scripture Reading
_____ Memory Verse _____ CR
_____ Encouragement
_____ Exercise
_____ Aerobic

_____ Strength
_____ Flexibility

DAY 5: Date _____

Morning _____

Midday _____

Evening _____

Snacks _____

_____ Meat ☐ Prayer
_____ Bread ☐ Bible Study
_____ Vegetable ☐ Scripture Reading
_____ Fruit ☐ Memory Verse
_____ Milk ☐ Encouragement
_____ Fat _____ Water

Exercise
Aerobic _____

Strength _____
Flexibility _____

DAY 6: Date _____

Morning _____

Midday _____

Evening _____

Snacks _____

_____ Meat ☐ Prayer
_____ Bread ☐ Bible Study
_____ Vegetable ☐ Scripture Reading
_____ Fruit ☐ Memory Verse
_____ Milk ☐ Encouragement
_____ Fat _____ Water

Exercise
Aerobic _____

Strength _____
Flexibility _____

DAY 7: Date _____

Morning _____

Midday _____

Evening _____

Snacks _____

_____ Meat ☐ Prayer
_____ Bread ☐ Bible Study
_____ Vegetable ☐ Scripture Reading
_____ Fruit ☐ Memory Verse
_____ Milk ☐ Encouragement
_____ Fat _____ Water

Exercise
Aerobic _____

Strength _____
Flexibility _____

DAY 1: Date _____

Morning _____

Midday _____

Evening _____

Snacks _____

___ Meat	☐ Prayer
___ Bread	☐ Bible Study
___ Vegetable	☐ Scripture Reading
___ Fruit	☐ Memory Verse
___ Milk	☐ Encouragement
___ Fat	___ Water

Exercise
Aerobic _____
Strength _____
Flexibility _____

DAY 2: Date _____

Morning _____

Midday _____

Evening _____

Snacks _____

___ Meat	☐ Prayer
___ Bread	☐ Bible Study
___ Vegetable	☐ Scripture Reading
___ Fruit	☐ Memory Verse
___ Milk	☐ Encouragement
___ Fat	___ Water

Exercise
Aerobic _____
Strength _____
Flexibility _____

DAY 3: Date _____

Morning _____

Midday _____

Evening _____

Snacks _____

___ Meat	☐ Prayer
___ Bread	☐ Bible Study
___ Vegetable	☐ Scripture Reading
___ Fruit	☐ Memory Verse
___ Milk	☐ Encouragement
___ Fat	___ Water

Exercise
Aerobic _____
Strength _____
Flexibility _____

DAY 4: Date _____

Morning _____

Midday _____

Evening _____

Snacks _____

___ Meat	☐ Prayer
___ Bread	☐ Bible Study
___ Vegetable	☐ Scripture Reading
___ Fruit	☐ Memory Verse
___ Milk	☐ Encouragement
___ Fat	___ Water

Exercise
Aerobic _____
Strength _____
Flexibility _____

FIRST PLACE CR

Name _____

Date _____ through _____

Week # _____ Calorie Level _____

Daily Exchange Plan

Level	Meat	Bread	Veggie	Fruit	Milk	Fat
1200	4-5	5-6	3	2-3	2-3	3-4
1400	5-6	6-7	3-4	3-4	2-3	3-4
1500	5-6	7-8	3-4	3-4	2-3	3-4
1600	6-7	8-9	3-4	3-4	2-3	3-4
1800	6-7	10-11	3-4	3-4	2-3	4-5
2000	6-7	11-12	4-5	4-5	2-3	4-5
2400	7-8	12-13	4-5	4-5	2-3	6-7
2600	8-9	13-14	4-5	4-5	2-3	7-8
2600	9-10	14-15	5	5	2-3	7-8
2800	9-10	15-16	5	5	2-3	9

You may always choose the high range of vegetables and fruits. Limit your high range selections to only one of the following: meat, bread, milk or fat.

___ Loss ___ Gain ___ Maintain
___ Attendance ___ Bible Study
___ Prayer ___ Scripture Reading
___ Memory Verse ___ CR
___ Encouragement
___ Exercise
Aerobic ___
Strength ___
Flexibility ___

DAY 5: Date _____

Morning _____

Midday _____

Evening _____

Snacks _____

___ Meat
___ Bread
___ Vegetable
___ Fruit
___ Milk
___ Fat
Exercise
Aerobic ___

☐ Prayer
☐ Bible Study
☐ Scripture Reading
☐ Memory Verse
☐ Encouragement
Water ___

Strength _____
Flexibility _____

DAY 6: Date _____

Morning _____

Midday _____

Evening _____

Snacks _____

___ Meat
___ Bread
___ Vegetable
___ Fruit
___ Milk
___ Fat
Exercise
Aerobic ___

☐ Prayer
☐ Bible Study
☐ Scripture Reading
☐ Memory Verse
☐ Encouragement
Water ___

Strength _____
Flexibility _____

DAY 7: Date _____

Morning _____

Midday _____

Evening _____

Snacks _____

___ Meat
___ Bread
___ Vegetable
___ Fruit
___ Milk
___ Fat
Exercise
Aerobic ___

☐ Prayer
☐ Bible Study
☐ Scripture Reading
☐ Memory Verse
☐ Encouragement
Water ___

Strength _____
Flexibility _____

DAY 1: Date _____

Morning _____

Midday _____

Evening _____

Snacks _____

____ Meat	☐ Prayer
____ Bread	☐ Bible Study
____ Vegetable	☐ Scripture Reading
____ Fruit	☐ Memory Verse
____ Milk	☐ Encouragement
____ Fat	____ Water

Exercise
Aerobic _____
Strength _____
Flexibility _____

DAY 2: Date _____

Morning _____

Midday _____

Evening _____

Snacks _____

____ Meat	☐ Prayer
____ Bread	☐ Bible Study
____ Vegetable	☐ Scripture Reading
____ Fruit	☐ Memory Verse
____ Milk	☐ Encouragement
____ Fat	____ Water

Exercise
Aerobic _____
Strength _____
Flexibility _____

DAY 3: Date _____

Morning _____

Midday _____

Evening _____

Snacks _____

____ Meat	☐ Prayer
____ Bread	☐ Bible Study
____ Vegetable	☐ Scripture Reading
____ Fruit	☐ Memory Verse
____ Milk	☐ Encouragement
____ Fat	____ Water

Exercise
Aerobic _____
Strength _____
Flexibility _____

DAY 4: Date _____

Morning _____

Midday _____

Evening _____

Snacks _____

____ Meat	☐ Prayer
____ Bread	☐ Bible Study
____ Vegetable	☐ Scripture Reading
____ Fruit	☐ Memory Verse
____ Milk	☐ Encouragement
____ Fat	____ Water

Exercise
Aerobic _____
Strength _____
Flexibility _____

FIRST PLACE CR

Name _____

Date _____ through _____

Week # _____ Calorie Level _____

Daily Exchange Plan

Level	Meat	Bread	Veggie	Fruit	Milk	Fat
1200	4-5	5-6	3	2-3	2-3	3-4
1400	5-6	6-7	3-4	3-4	2-3	3-4
1500	5-6	7-8	3-4	3-4	2-3	3-4
1600	6-7	8-9	3-4	3-4	2-3	3-4
1800	6-7	10-11	3-4	3-4	2-3	4-5
2000	6-7	11-12	4-5	4-5	2-3	4-5
2200	7-8	12-13	4-5	4-5	2-3	6-7
2400	8-9	13-14	4-5	4-5	2-3	7-8
2600	9-10	14-15	5	5	2-3	7-8
2800	9-10	15-16	5	5	2-3	9

You may always choose the high range of vegetables and fruits. Limit your high range selections to only one of the following: meat, bread, milk or fat.

_____ Loss _____ Gain _____ Maintain

_____ Attendance _____ Bible Study
_____ Prayer _____ Scripture Reading
_____ Memory Verse _____ CR
_____ Encouragement
_____ Exercise
Aerobic _____

Strength _____
Flexibility _____

DAY 5: Date _____

Morning _____

Midday _____

Evening _____

Snacks _____

_____ Meat   ☐ Prayer
_____ Bread   ☐ Bible Study
_____ Vegetable ☐ Scripture Reading
_____ Fruit   ☐ Memory Verse
_____ Milk   ☐ Encouragement
_____ Fat   ☐ Water

Exercise
Aerobic _____

Strength _____
Flexibility _____

DAY 6: Date _____

Morning _____

Midday _____

Evening _____

Snacks _____

_____ Meat   ☐ Prayer
_____ Bread   ☐ Bible Study
_____ Vegetable ☐ Scripture Reading
_____ Fruit   ☐ Memory Verse
_____ Milk   ☐ Encouragement
_____ Fat   ☐ Water

Exercise
Aerobic _____

Strength _____
Flexibility _____

DAY 7: Date _____

Morning _____

Midday _____

Evening _____

Snacks _____

_____ Meat   ☐ Prayer
_____ Bread   ☐ Bible Study
_____ Vegetable ☐ Scripture Reading
_____ Fruit   ☐ Memory Verse
_____ Milk   ☐ Encouragement
_____ Fat   ☐ Water

Exercise
Aerobic _____

Strength _____
Flexibility _____

DAY 1: Date _____

Morning _____

Midday _____

Evening _____

Snacks _____

___ Meat	☐ Prayer
___ Bread	☐ Bible Study
___ Vegetable	☐ Scripture Reading
___ Fruit	☐ Memory Verse
___ Milk	☐ Encouragement
___ Fat	___ Water

Exercise
Aerobic _____
Strength _____
Flexibility _____

DAY 2: Date _____

Morning _____

Midday _____

Evening _____

Snacks _____

___ Meat	☐ Prayer
___ Bread	☐ Bible Study
___ Vegetable	☐ Scripture Reading
___ Fruit	☐ Memory Verse
___ Milk	☐ Encouragement
___ Fat	___ Water

Exercise
Aerobic _____
Strength _____
Flexibility _____

DAY 3: Date _____

Morning _____

Midday _____

Evening _____

Snacks _____

___ Meat	☐ Prayer
___ Bread	☐ Bible Study
___ Vegetable	☐ Scripture Reading
___ Fruit	☐ Memory Verse
___ Milk	☐ Encouragement
___ Fat	___ Water

Exercise
Aerobic _____
Strength _____
Flexibility _____

DAY 4: Date _____

Morning _____

Midday _____

Evening _____

Snacks _____

___ Meat	☐ Prayer
___ Bread	☐ Bible Study
___ Vegetable	☐ Scripture Reading
___ Fruit	☐ Memory Verse
___ Milk	☐ Encouragement
___ Fat	___ Water

Exercise
Aerobic _____
Strength _____
Flexibility _____

Name _____

Date _____ through _____

Week # _____ Calorie Level _____

Daily Exchange Plan

Level	Meat	Bread	Veggie	Fruit	Milk	Fat
1200	4-5	5-6	3	2-3	2-3	3-4
1400	5-6	6-7	3-4	3-4	2-3	3-4
1500	5-6	7-8	3-4	3-4	2-3	3-4
1600	6-7	8-9	3-4	3-4	2-3	3-4
1800	6-7	10-11	3-4	3-4	2-3	4-5
2000	6-7	11-12	4-5	4-5	2-3	4-5
2200	7-8	12-13	4-5	4-5	2-3	6-7
2400	8-9	13-14	4-5	4-5	2-3	7-8
2600	9-10	14-15	5	5	2-3	7-8
2800	9-10	15-16	5	5	2-3	9

You may always choose the high range of vegetables and fruits. Limit your high range selections to only one of the following: meat, bread, milk or fat.

_____ Loss _____ Gain _____ Maintain

_____ Attendance _____ Bible Study
_____ Prayer _____ Scripture Reading
_____ Memory Verse _____ CR
_____ Encouragement
_____ Exercise
_____ Aerobic

_____ Strength
_____ Flexibility

DAY 5: Date _____

Morning _____

Midday _____

Evening _____

Snacks _____

_____ Meat ☐ Prayer
_____ Bread ☐ Bible Study
_____ Vegetable ☐ Scripture Reading
_____ Fruit ☐ Memory Verse
_____ Milk ☐ Encouragement
_____ Fat ☐ Water

Exercise
Aerobic _____

Strength _____
Flexibility _____

DAY 6: Date _____

Morning _____

Midday _____

Evening _____

Snacks _____

_____ Meat ☐ Prayer
_____ Bread ☐ Bible Study
_____ Vegetable ☐ Scripture Reading
_____ Fruit ☐ Memory Verse
_____ Milk ☐ Encouragement
_____ Fat ☐ Water

Exercise
Aerobic _____

Strength _____
Flexibility _____

DAY 7: Date _____

Morning _____

Midday _____

Evening _____

Snacks _____

_____ Meat ☐ Prayer
_____ Bread ☐ Bible Study
_____ Vegetable ☐ Scripture Reading
_____ Fruit ☐ Memory Verse
_____ Milk ☐ Encouragement
_____ Fat ☐ Water

Exercise
Aerobic _____

Strength _____
Flexibility _____

DAY 1: Date _____

Morning _____

Midday _____

Evening _____

Snacks _____

___ Meat	☐ Prayer
___ Bread	☐ Bible Study
___ Vegetable	☐ Scripture Reading
___ Fruit	☐ Memory Verse
___ Milk	☐ Encouragement
___ Fat ___ Water	

Exercise

Aerobic _____

Strength _____

Flexibility _____

DAY 2: Date _____

Morning _____

Midday _____

Evening _____

Snacks _____

___ Meat	☐ Prayer
___ Bread	☐ Bible Study
___ Vegetable	☐ Scripture Reading
___ Fruit	☐ Memory Verse
___ Milk	☐ Encouragement
___ Fat ___ Water	

Exercise

Aerobic _____

Strength _____

Flexibility _____

DAY 3: Date _____

Morning _____

Midday _____

Evening _____

Snacks _____

___ Meat	☐ Prayer
___ Bread	☐ Bible Study
___ Vegetable	☐ Scripture Reading
___ Fruit	☐ Memory Verse
___ Milk	☐ Encouragement
___ Fat ___ Water	

Exercise

Aerobic _____

Strength _____

Flexibility _____

DAY 4: Date _____

Morning _____

Midday _____

Evening _____

Snacks _____

___ Meat	☐ Prayer
___ Bread	☐ Bible Study
___ Vegetable	☐ Scripture Reading
___ Fruit	☐ Memory Verse
___ Milk	☐ Encouragement
___ Fat ___ Water	

Exercise

Aerobic _____

Strength _____

Flexibility _____

FIRST PLACE CR

Name _____

Date _____ through _____

Week # _____ Calorie Level _____

Daily Exchange Plan

Level	Meat	Bread	Veggie	Fruit	Milk	Fat
1200	4-5	5-6	3	2-3	2-3	3-4
1400	5-6	6-7	3-4	3-4	2-3	3-4
1500	5-6	7-8	3-4	3-4	2-3	3-4
1600	6-7	8-9	3-4	3-4	2-3	3-4
1800	6-7	10-11	3-4	3-4	2-3	4-5
2000	6-7	11-12	4-5	4-5	2-3	4-5
2200	7-8	12-13	4-5	4-5	2-3	6-7
2400	8-9	13-14	4-5	4-5	2-3	7-8
2600	9-10	14-15	5	5	2-3	7-8
2800	9-10	15-16	5	5	2-3	9

You may always choose the high range of vegetables and fruits. Limit your high range selections to only one of the following: meat, bread, milk or fat.

_____ Loss _____ Gain _____ Maintain

___ Attendance ___ Bible Study
___ Prayer ___ Scripture Reading
___ Memory Verse ___ CR
___ Encouragement
___ Exercise
Aerobic _____

Strength _____
Flexibility _____

DAY 7: Date _____

Morning _____
_____

Midday _____
_____

Evening _____
_____

Snacks _____
_____

_____ Meat 　　☐ Prayer
_____ Bread 　　☐ Bible Study
_____ Vegetable 　☐ Scripture Reading
_____ Fruit 　　☐ Memory Verse
_____ Milk 　　☐ Encouragement
_____ Fat 　　Water _____

Exercise
Aerobic _____

Strength _____
Flexibility _____

DAY 6: Date _____

Morning _____
_____

Midday _____
_____

Evening _____
_____

Snacks _____
_____

_____ Meat 　　☐ Prayer
_____ Bread 　　☐ Bible Study
_____ Vegetable 　☐ Scripture Reading
_____ Fruit 　　☐ Memory Verse
_____ Milk 　　☐ Encouragement
_____ Fat 　　Water _____

Exercise
Aerobic _____

Strength _____
Flexibility _____

DAY 5: Date _____

Morning _____
_____

Midday _____
_____

Evening _____
_____

Snacks _____
_____

_____ Meat 　　☐ Prayer
_____ Bread 　　☐ Bible Study
_____ Vegetable 　☐ Scripture Reading
_____ Fruit 　　☐ Memory Verse
_____ Milk 　　☐ Encouragement
_____ Fat 　　Water _____

Exercise
Aerobic _____

Strength _____
Flexibility _____

DAY 1: Date _____

Morning _____

Midday _____

Evening _____

Snacks _____

____ Meat	☐ Prayer
____ Bread	☐ Bible Study
____ Vegetable	☐ Scripture Reading
____ Fruit	☐ Memory Verse
____ Milk	☐ Encouragement
____ Fat	____ Water

Exercise

Aerobic _____

Strength _____

Flexibility _____

DAY 2: Date _____

Morning _____

Midday _____

Evening _____

Snacks _____

____ Meat	☐ Prayer
____ Bread	☐ Bible Study
____ Vegetable	☐ Scripture Reading
____ Fruit	☐ Memory Verse
____ Milk	☐ Encouragement
____ Fat	____ Water

Exercise

Aerobic _____

Strength _____

Flexibility _____

DAY 3: Date _____

Morning _____

Midday _____

Evening _____

Snacks _____

____ Meat	☐ Prayer
____ Bread	☐ Bible Study
____ Vegetable	☐ Scripture Reading
____ Fruit	☐ Memory Verse
____ Milk	☐ Encouragement
____ Fat	____ Water

Exercise

Aerobic _____

Strength _____

Flexibility _____

DAY 4: Date _____

Morning _____

Midday _____

Evening _____

Snacks _____

____ Meat	☐ Prayer
____ Bread	☐ Bible Study
____ Vegetable	☐ Scripture Reading
____ Fruit	☐ Memory Verse
____ Milk	☐ Encouragement
____ Fat	____ Water

Exercise

Aerobic _____

Strength _____

Flexibility _____